BIRTH IN AWARENESS

A Handbook of Prenatal Yoga

GABRIELLE EARLS

Book Website
www.birthinawareness.com.au

Give feedback on the book at: gabrielle.earls@gmail.com

Praise for *Birth in Awareness*

"Gabrielle Earls has blessed us with her book *Birth in Awareness*. It is so very useful, practical and well done, that it makes my heart sing! Folded in these pages is a perfect blend of the essential *nature* of yoga for mothers, the *science/anatomy* of benefits, plus balancing of *spirit*. Gabrielle brings her Doula skills to light by making the "How to" so clear that mothers and teachers of yoga feel guided and supported in their practice. The illustrations are simply wonderful. I am astonished."

Robin Lim ~ Midwife, Doula, Grandmother
March 2017, dawn, Bali, Indonesia

"Finally a comprehensive book on prenatal yoga which will add value to any dedicated prenatal yoga teacher or those teaching general classes with little options to offer for the occasional pregnant student. Gabby has made all the information any yoga teacher should know easily accessible, with beautiful illustrations and clear and precise explanation, without losing the depth of yoga. I would take it further and say that even Doulas, midwives and other healthcare professionals working with pregnant women will get something valuable out of this book."

Dini Martinez ~ Prenatal yoga teacher, Doula, mother of three)

"In this gem of a read, Gabrielle offers us not only an interesting and informative handbook to navigate pregnancy, yoga and birthing for yoga teachers but also a supportive roadmap for a mother-to-be on her journey. Her own fascinating story is part of the wisdom she offers, and yet she has an incredible ability to see everyone's journey and practice as unique and their own. I've been blessed to have her input on many of my Yin Yoga teacher trainings since she herself took the course. If you cannot have her advice or support in person – then this is the next best thing!"

Mel Mclaughlin ~ The Yin Space

Contents

Preface

When I gave birth for the first time over ten years ago, I went into a state of shock at how different the birth was to any of my expectations. It seems I had not been ready for labour. I thought I had been prepared for the physical intensity but as contractions strengthened and the medical interventions started I was out of my depth. I had also not been prepared for the upheaval I experienced physically, mentally and spiritually when I became a mother. The realisation of responsibility after my son's birth; the tiredness, demands and newness of having a baby both surprised me and changed me.

I felt traumatised because the birth did not work out how I planned, and this led me on a journey of self-discovery and healing through yoga. I turned my back on everything I had known, shutting down that life of striving to succeed and achieve. I booked a one way ticket to Thailand to study yoga.

My baby grew into a boy over the years we spent in Thailand, India, Nicaragua, Guatemala and Peru. I had a deep yearning to understand how I could have gotten it so wrong, when in most other areas of my life, I achieved and succeeded in what I set out to do.

I thought if I learned everything I could find about birth and yoga, I could understand how it happened. What I ended up studying was myself.

When I started to teach prenatal yoga and doula (supporting people give birth), I focused on what I needed to do to help others. My intention was to support women so they did not have to go through what I did. So that they could get the birth they wanted... if they just knew the right things and were more prepared than I had been.

When my second son was born seven years later, I knew everything I thought I needed to know. Of course the birth went nothing as planned. I tore an intercostal muscle as my waters broke and I could not breathe properly or move without experiencing pain.

Through this painful and challenging 48 hours, I had an expectation that I had to get it right. I was a doula and yoga teacher and knew what to do; this belief set off a raging internal battle.

The shift came not from what I knew about birth or yoga, but what I knew about myself. I accessed a part of me so deep that I found a way to let go of that expectation by accepting the situation as it was. From there, I surrendered into the moment, and my baby was born soon after.

I have realised that we can't guarantee—even if someone comes to our birthing and yoga classes—that they will have the birth that they want. Nor can we promise that their birth will be tranquil and calm if they learn the right things. Instead, we open up the possibilities of coping and experiencing their birth in an aware way. We can add to their own inner journey of self discovery as preparation for the trip of a lifetime.

Birth is raw and primal. Through birth, what we think we know or have is stripped away and the depths of the self are accessed. Through the yoga practice, we offer a space to go inside to build up self-awareness, courage, strength and determination. We prepare people to birth in the moment and do what needs doing along each step of their journey.

This book has been inspired by the different practices I have learned from my travels. It has stemmed from inspiring midwives, yoga teachers, doulas, mothers and many other people I have worked with and taught with over the years.

This is a guide on practices that lead people within, so I hope it can help you discover more about yourself.

Gabrielle Earls
Sydney, Australia

Chapter ONE

Prenatal Yoga

Prenatal Yoga

As I booked a ski trip with my family, I reflected on my first pregnancy ten years ago. At that point I had never had a baby. Skiing was something completely new and unknown to me, as pregnancy and birth was back then. As I watched movies of people skiing, I realised that getting on the slopes needs preparation, just as moving through pregnancy and readying for birth takes preparation.

The first time I gave birth, I expected it to be quite easy. Billions of people have done it over the ages... and the human race is thriving. As I sat in the space between the idea of skiing in my head and actually skiing, I could see the parallels with birthing.

I heard from other people about their ski experiences and found out what happened to them the first time they skied, listened to great stories and horror stories about skiing. Yet, I had no real idea of how I would ski until I got to the slopes. Then I needed to stay in the moment, as skiing takes full effort and concentration.

I squatted and built strength, and practised moving my hips while staying relaxed through my body. I took it breath-by-breath and faced my fears as I prepared to shoot down the mountain at high speeds. People have died skiing; they have also had the most exhilarating moments of their lives. We don't know in advance what the snow will be like that day, or the weather, or so many other variables that will all add to the experience. Just like birth.

There are so many stories out there, so much information available about birth and how to prepare. We are in an information age. Google can answer almost any question. There are books, courses, informative blogs, apps and conferences on birth and how to give birth. We can watch women giving birth on a live stream on Facebook.

We can pick the information we want, yet until labour begins we don't know how it will be or how we will cope. For labour to fully establish, our thinking brain needs to move out of the way and all that information gathered goes with it. It is what is inside each of us that Google can't answer. This stays as we give birth. There are ways we can access this deep resource and explore ourselves in preparation for the journey. The prenatal yoga practice is one of those ways.

Each pregnancy and birth is unique for every woman. Every day around the world about 350,000 babies are born.[1]

Although we can't prepare expectant parents for a particular type of birth, as there are so many variables, we can invite deep internal connection with the life growing inside. We can invite space to accept the unexpected.

When I was studying to become a Doula, I spent a month in a small village in rural Guatemala assisting an indigenous midwife. After one of the births, we were given two live chickens to carry on our walk back home. These were part of the payment! It was such a different scenario than I was used to at home. Yet, the way this beautiful mama's body worked through labour was unique for her while going through the same physiological processes. The midwife I lived and worked with has given birth to thirteen of her own babies and has been present at hundreds of births. She told me that each of those pregnancies and births were unique and unpredictable in the way they unfolded. Indeed, she believes that each birth happens exactly as it needs to.

The Prenatal Yoga Practice

The prenatal yoga practice offers a nurturing time of self exploration while encouraging the body, mind and spirit to open and embrace the transformations of pregnancy and birth.

Through a prenatal yoga practice there is time and space to build up confidence in the self and the body. It allows for surprise about what is possible; what one can do when focused and concentrating.

Pregnant women know their bodies best, and so intuition is cultivated during pregnancy. If something doesn't feel right to them, they need to learn to trust and fully listen to that intuitive voice. The deep inner listening is a great practice for the months of birth preparation, as well as for labour, where women have to go deeply within.

Incorporated in the prenatal yoga practice are asanas, pranayama, mindfulness and deep relaxation. These practices offer ways to see ourselves—our reactions, responses and emotions in the moment—without becoming attached. Through the practices, women will be releasing expectation of the self and of how things should be, while building skills of being present and accepting of what is in the moment. These are all powerful ways to support pregnancy, labour and birth.

As we know, although it sounds simple, staying in the moment, each moment, and being present, takes a lot of work in regular life. In birth, there are the sensations of labour and contractions, hormones, unfamiliar environments and unexpected events to contend with. This can make it even more challenging at times and can push women to their limits and beyond.

Through the practices, women learn how to interrupt suffering, rather than trying to end all pain. In labour, the only way to end pain is from an epidural. How one responds to the pain is the choice. Learning ways to 'dive in' and find ways to experience what is going on, without suffering, is a key element in prenatal yoga and in birth.

asana (the physical practice)

Women's bodies are in a continual state of change in pregnancy; something that felt wonderful one week may not work for them the next. Some asana may be easier for pregnant women, with the added help of increased relaxin. Others may be more challenging, due to the added weight of the baby. Nausea and lightheadedness may get in the way, and so the practice will need to be adjusted according to how the practitioner perceives the woman's comfort level at the time.

For all women at some point, labour is intense, just as yoga practice has moments of intensity. It may be from the asana one day... or being unable to stay focused on the breath another day. Women face different levels of intensity with different asana and practices. Exactly what point the intensity will occur for each person is near impossible to predict. By getting used to not knowing this level, on any particular day one can prepare both mentally and physically to take the path as it unfolds, with all of its unexpected turns, in an aware and non-reactive way.

Child's pose is often a good option for taking rest if women are feeling too challenged. This is more commonly needed in a general class when giving a pregnant student modifications.

Props can be helpful in a prenatal practice and these can include walls, chairs, bolsters, blocks and folded blankets.

pranayama (the breath)

Breath awareness, and engaging the diaphragm while breathing, are both important elements for birth preparation. In labour, women often find it easier to exhale through their mouths. At times in the yoga practice, exhaling through the mouth may also be better for them. If the breath becomes strained, listen to that and reduce intensity.

drishti (concentration)

Prenatal yoga can be practised with eyes opened or closed—which is another way to prepare for the physical side of birth. There will be times when people will need eyes wide open, and other times that the darkness and space within calls. Often I find that pregnant women usually need their eyes open for balance.

The Space

Women have approximately one extra litre of blood circulating through their bodies through pregnancy,[2] which increases their body temperature. It is usual for a pregnant woman's body to be slightly warmer than normal. If you are heating the space or teach in a hot climate, be aware of how warm the room becomes. With too much heat, pregnant women can feel nauseous and uncomfortable.

Chapter TWO

Pregnancy

Traditionally, pregnancy is made up of three trimesters. New ways of thinking suggest that there are actually four trimesters. The first three are when the baby is developing within and is covered in this chapter. The fourth trimester is the early postpartum time and is explored in the postpartum chapter.

First Trimester

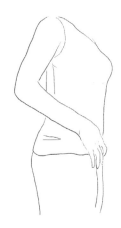

The first trimester is from week one to twelve of a pregnancy. It's a time for women to start embracing the transformation and changes that pregnancy brings. It can be an anxious time for some, especially those who may have had a previous miscarriage.

I found out I was pregnant with my second son the day after we landed in Nepal for a 3 week trip. We were going to visit Kathmandu and trek on the Annapurna circuit trail. I found the motion and the unfamiliar smells to be very unsettling. I was particularly challenged by the altitude when we trekked. I also worried about the hygiene aspects and so was very particular about what I ate on that journey and where the food was prepared.

Through the first trimester, it is recommended that anyone new to yoga rest and wait until their second trimester before embarking on a prenatal asana practice. Regular students can keep practising, with modifications, although often the nausea from morning sickness and tiredness sees women pulling back from their regular practice until the second trimester.

Sometimes what is most needed in the first trimester is space for deep relaxation and permission to take it easy.

Physical and emotional considerations for women in the beginning of their pregnancy are listed in the table below.

Physical	Emotional
Often do not look obviously pregnant.	Moody from the hormone changes.
May feel nauseated.	Worry about how life is going to change.
Altered sense of smell.	Worry about the baby and if it is healthy, particularly if there is a history of miscarriage.
Feeling tired and less energetic.	It is generally a secret as the norm is for people to reveal they are pregnant after the first trimester. People try to act normal even though a huge change is going on inside.
Swelling of breasts and they may feel sore and tender.	
Increased need to urinate.	

Second Trimester

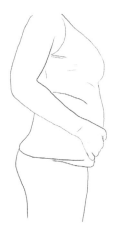

The second trimester goes from weeks 13 to 26 of pregnancy and is traditionally when pregnancy news is shared with friends and family.

The second trimester is typically the highest energy part of pregnancy and the time women start or resume an asana practice.

Women generally have a healthier diet in pregnancy, and if they drank or socialised a lot pre-pregnancy, then this generally curbs. People tend to find sleep easier and deeper in this trimester—although this is not always the case—as the body has not yet become too uncomfortable. Some women in this trimester have told me that they feel healthier and more energetic than they have ever felt.

Physical and emotional considerations for this stage of pregnancy can include the following:

Physical	Emotional
Women start gaining weight and looking pregnant. Second time mothers will generally show earlier.	Feelings of being more balanced and energised.
Veins in the legs and breasts may begin to pop out from the increased blood supply and pregnancy hormones.	Shifting emotions as the pregnancy becomes more obvious to people looking in.

Physical	Emotional
The uterus has moved up and isn't pressing onto the bladder as much so the need to urinate decreases.	Excitement of feeling the baby's heart beat.
The nausea generally stops or lessens.	Fear that the baby is OK. There is typically an ultrasound performed at 20 weeks to check the health of the baby.
Might feel warmer from the extra blood supply.	Excitement or disappointment if they have found out the sex of the baby and it is/is not what they were wanting/expecting.
Physical balance can start to be affected as the uterus grows.	Anxious if waiting for test results from the ultrasound.
Around week 20 the baby's kicks can start to be felt.	
Might start getting stretch marks.	
There is a 20 week scan which determines any abnormalities or potential issues. People can also choose to find out the sex of their baby.	

Third Trimester

The third trimester is from weeks 27 to 40 and above.

In the third trimester, women may prefer to do less asana and more relaxation practices, especially if they are feeling heavier and more tired. The build-up of the relaxin hormone in the body also influences the

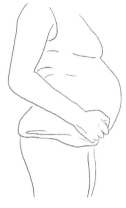

joints and so it is important at this stage not to overstretch.

Visits to midwife, GP or obstetrician become more frequent. Talk of induction can begin if there are any reasons for this. Women with gestational diabetes or particularly small babies may also be induced. Blood pressure is monitored to keep an eye out for any signs of hypertension.

Physical	Emotional
May feel even more tired.	Generally women are more emotional than the second trimester.
Aches and pains in the belly and back are more common.	There may be anxiety about the birth.
May have pains in the top of the legs and pelvis from the stretching ligaments.	A time of nesting and getting things ready for baby.
May develop heartburn.	Often feelings of excitement arise about meeting their baby soon.
May start to develop breathlessness closer to the end of the pregnancy.	Emotional outbursts influenced by the flux of hormones as birth nears.
Baby may drop down and release the lungs but increase pressure again on the bladder.	
May experience Braxton Hicks contractions.	

When women ask: 'until when in my pregnancy can I practise pre-natal yoga?', my general response is 'through birth'!

A few years ago, a student came to a pre-natal class in early labour. She did the asana practice, resting when needed, moving with her contractions. She then went home to continue her labour, giving birth that evening. Even if women are not coming to a class through labour, the different asana and practices can be used through till birth.

Development of the Fetus

Pregnancy and birth are times of great transformation for a woman as she evolves from maiden to mother. The development from conception to birth of a human being is equally transformational. In 2016, scientists discovered that there is a flash of light when the sperm meets the ovum.[3]

From the moment the sperm and ovum connect, there is transformation as the cells start to divide and create human life. In fertilisation, the sperm contributes DNA. Everything else that makes up the cell comes from the ovum. Due to this, the energy of each person at conception comes from the feminine, through the mitochondria. The mitochondria are the energy centres of cells and of life. These structures are sometimes described as 'cellular power plants' because they generate most of the cell's supply of adenosine triphosphate (ATP), used as a source of chemical energy.[4] As soon as the blastocyst—which is the ball of cells—attaches to the uterine wall, chemicals are secreted to signal the mother's body to start changing. Ovulation ceases, her breasts begin to grow and the uterine wall softens.[5]

The embryo also goes through significant transformations. During the second week of its life, a dark mark appears on the back of the embryo which marks the position of the spinal cord. By the end of the third week the heart has begun to beat. Although the embryo will be only be approximately 4 mm, weighing less than a gram by the sixth week, all the major organs have started forming. The embryo is known as the fetus from week eight until birth.

By 14 weeks the fetus is fully formed and very active, although the movements generally can't be felt. For the first half of pregnancy, major developments are taking place with the fetus while the mother's body is gently preparing for accommodating the needs of the growing baby.

At 18 weeks, the fetus' tastebuds have begun to develop on their tongue and as the tiny bones inside the ears begin to harden they begin to hear sounds such as their mother's voice, heart beat and even digestion. The lungs are also developing, however, the baby will receive oxygen via the placenta until born. After another month of development, at week 22, women will feel their fetus moving inside, which is such a unique sensation. The fetus' heartbeat can be heard with stethoscopes and they are sensitive to touch.

At 26 weeks, the patterns of the brainwaves now resemble those of a full-term newborn child. By week 30, the fetus has begun to control their own body temperature and its bone marrow has completely taken over responsibility for the production of red blood cells.

By week 34, the fetus is perfectly formed and the proportions are as you would expect them to be at birth. From there, the fetus grows, and as he or she prepares for birth, the lungs mature and the last of the fat is laid down.[6]

There are many detailed resources available on the development of the fetus at each stage, including week-by-week updates you can be emailed and apps that pictorially show the fetus' development.

Opening to Pregnancy and Birth

Opening to different ideas with visualisations through pregnancy are a good way to prepare for labour and birth. On one level, visualising the stages of pregnancy and the changes within are key. On a deeper level, there is opening of the woman to her transformation through birth, thus preparing to open to the intensity of labour by softening into the flow of contractions.

Each contraction, whether spontaneous or induced, works on opening and release. If contractions stall during labour or do not function fully to open through the cervix, these meditations can be a powerful way to bring that focus on opening back.

A practice to open with each breath

Inhale and feel the space the breath is creating. As you exhale, feel yourself move into that space. Follow each breath without controlling the breath. Open through the body on the inhalation and soften, release and let go on the exhalation.

Breath by breath, follow your rhythm and soften into your flow of breath. As your breath deepens naturally as you relax, your body opens and releases. Breathe in to open and expand. Breathe out to release and let go.

Use this breath throughout a practice. In an asana, focus on where the body is opening and being stretched, and use each breath as a way to work with the posture. For birth this works equally well. Focus on taking the contractions breath-by-breath and on opening to the intensity; even focus on the open feeling that the contraction is creating within.

An opening meditation

As you close your eyes, open the mouth and release the jaw by moving it from side to side. As you do this, be aware of release through the perineum.

If you are clenching your hands into a fist, open through the hands

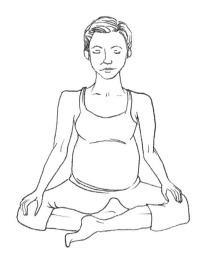

and relax your fingers, release any tension through your fingers and hands, and feel that release up through your wrists and arms. Be aware of your toes and gently move through the toes to fully release through each toe.

With your body now completely relaxed, take your awareness to your heart centre. That space in your chest that you feel expanding and opening. With a very subtle movement, draw your shoulder blades in towards each other and as you do this, feel your heart open even more.

Each time you inhale, be aware of the opening through your chest and your heart space. Each time you exhale, soften into that space and as you soften, your heart space will open even more.

Breath by breath, you open and expand. Through your body there is opening and expansion. As you open through your body you open through your mind, and there are endless possibilities.

With each breath you open more... opening to the changes through your body through pregnancy... opening to the changes that having a baby is making to you and your life. Keep opening with each breath.

Chapter THREE

Letting Go

In prenatal yoga, the question for practitioners is often not 'what can my body do or not do', but rather 'how much can I let go?' The sensations and shifts that the asana and breath work allow builds awareness, and so surrender can be a spontaneous process.

Letting go through pregnancy and birth has many layers; from the decided and completely conscious release to the unexpected and spontaneous release. Through the yoga practice, emotions can often be released as parts of the body are released through breath and movement. This is why people can experience a spontaneous emotional outburst in a yoga practice. As teachers holding the space, it is important to witness and be aware of the releases without interfering.

There are many other ways of letting go. It may be letting go of expectations of their bodies if they don't seem to be doing exactly what they want. An experienced practitioner may not be able to move her body into positions that were once easy. A new practitioner may find the sensations difficult to deal with as she moves through the practice. Someone may not be able to get their body into the shape of the woman next to them, who seems to be so much more flexible. Someone else may be letting go of an argument she had a couple of years ago with her partner that never fully resolved. There may be a release of resentment from deep within their tissues from childhood that may not be consciously remembered.

It could be letting go of reactions to physical sensations. Practising downward-facing dog may reveal pain in the back of the legs or discomfort elsewhere that wasn't there pre-pregnancy. She may have a cold and each movement makes everything ache. Her baby or placenta may be in a contraindicated position, or there may even be a medical condition that restricts the asana a woman is able to do through pregnancy.

An understanding of the koshas helps explain how subtle shifts can affect the entire being. For example, how a release through the physical body in a yoga practice can unleash a strong emotional release. Or how breathing with awareness can allow for a shift in a way of thinking.

The koshas are the layers surrounding the soul of a person. There are physical, subtle and causal bodies included in the layers of the koshas and these can be visualised like the layers of an onion. The layers are outlined in the table below.

Kosha	Sustained by	Body	
Annamaya	food	physical	Jivatman
Pranamaya	energy	subtle	
Manomaya	mind	subtle	SOUL
Vijnamaya	intellect	subtle	
Anandamaya	bliss	causal	

The emotions, mind and intellect can all affect the physical body and vice versa. For example, a person suffering from body pain carries this with them through the mind. Their emotions can be affected; they may have a shorter temper as they are trying to cope with the pain. They may be obsessed with thoughts of the pain in their mind. The opposite is also possible. Emotions that are out of balance or not freely expressed can manifest as physical blockages and pain in the body.

Unbalances through pregnancy and birth can build up through the koshas. If fear is not freely expressed, this may appear in the physical body as tightness through a muscle. Stretching in a yoga class may release the tightness and with that, an emotional release spontaneously follows. This is an example of how one layer can affect one or more other layers.

Being unable to let go of intellectual pursuits to make space for the pregnancy and birth can create an unbalance through the koshas. From this attempted 'mind control' comes tension through the body. Often this shows up as tension through the jaw from clenching, as well as tension through the upper shoulders.

In pregnancy, there is an additional set of koshas developing within the one body, more if there are multiple babies within. Something to think about is that there are hormones secreted into the bloodstream whenever the person experiences emotional reactions and responses. The mother's blood carries nutrients through the placenta to the fetus inside. Whatever hormones flow through the mother cross over into the baby. So, every emotion felt by the mother is experienced by the baby... every build up and also every release.

Letting Go of Expectations

Women can be heavily influenced by birthing stories from other women and may base their beliefs about birth on those stories. The stories may come from friends or family who had experiences that left trauma, and so the pregnant woman may carry fear that her birth will also turn out this way. If a friend had a quick birth, the woman may have expectation that to get it right, she too should also have a fast birth. This belief can manifest through the physical, emotional and spiritual layers of a person and influence how they labour and give birth.

Sometimes, women think they have to birth a certain way to belong to their social group. In some parts of Mexico there is a cesarean rate of 90%. Women wanting to birth naturally have to work hard against the social norm of cesarean birth to be able to even attempt a vaginal delivery.

In some subcultures around the world, natural easy birth is seen as the ideal and if you birth that way then you have done it right. Thus, difficult and long labours can be judged and so women might feel that they need to hide their story. All births are transformational, intense, life changing and to be admired. There is a huge transformation for mother, baby, family, and even society with the birth of each baby. Releasing ideas of an ideal birth, and being aware more deeply through birth, can heavily reduce birth trauma.

Practising prenatal yoga prepares a woman to be 'present' through their pregnancy, labour and birth. Instead of focusing on doing anything right, she builds her awareness of each moment as it rises, and continues this with the next and the next and the next. It takes bravery and a leap into the unknown to be able to let go, to access parts of themselves she may have never known before.

Letting Go through Labour

Through labour, it may be about letting go of the breath and not holding the breath to try to hold off the painful sensations. It may involve letting go of any tension through the jaw. There is a smooth muscle connection from the jaw down to the perineum. I have heard people comment that "a tight jaw makes a tight vagina." Ina May Gaskin, creator of *The Farm midwifery centre* has spoken of this idea. Loosening through the jaw releases through the body.

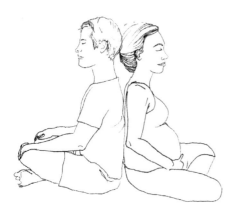

Physical, mental and emotional releases can all open up a woman in pregnancy and through birth.

We shift the focus from trying into allowing; from resisting into softening.

A practice to let go

Benefits

Deeply connective meditation. Can be practised through pregnancy, labour and post birth.

How to

Sit back-to-back with your partner and close your eyes. Feel the shared space between you. With neither partner controlling the breath or the rhythm, feel each others' breath as you connect back to back. Let your breaths flow together and as you relax into the shared space, notice how your breaths work and flow in sync together. With that aware-ness of breath, become the shared breath. Place concentration on each breath. As you sit together be aware of the breaths you are also sharing with your fetus inside.

Vocalising to let go

Sometimes there is the need to make sounds and express through vocalising. It can be releasing and supportive at times during labour to sync the sounds with a partner, just ensure to let go of any control while doing this.

On each inhale, take in a fresh breath and energy, expanding through the lungs and diaphragm.

AAAAAHHHHHH
OOOOOOHHHHHHHHH
AAAAAHHHHHH
OOOOOOHHHHHHHHH
AAAAAHHHHHH
OOOOOOHHHHHHHHH
AAAAAHHHHHH
OOOOOOHHHHHHHHH

Keep repeating this cycle with your in and out breath, in sync with your partner. Do 10 cycles of breath or as many as you like.

Chapter FOUR

Physiology of Labour and Birth

The Physiology of Labour and Birth

Physiology is the study of the function of the human body while hormones are what regulates the function of various body systems.[7] From the moment of conception through to approximately six months post birth, the hormonal system undergoes vast changes. Through pregnancy these changes have a great effect on a woman, and so yoga practice can assist these hormones.

Throughout pregnancy the changes in levels of relaxin, progesterone and oestrogen affects the body and emotions. Progesterone prepares the uterus for the implantation of the fetus. It can also positively affect stress. Increased oestrogen, which is associated with both positive and negative changes in mood and sex drive, also stimulates the growth of the uterus and improves blood flow between the uterus and placenta. Oestrogen peaks just before birth and declines afterward. Relaxin affects the flexibility of the connective tissues by softening them in preparation for birth.[8]

For quite some time, it was believed that it is the hormones from the fetus' lungs that signals their lungs are mature and ready to breathe once outside the body. When this happened, labour would commence. It was only recently that Australian researchers discovered a protein that the mother's body produces[9], which releases a 'safety switch', allowing the uterus to contract in a way that any stretched muscle should. Once this is released, the muscles are able to start contracting and releasing, which starts labour. What causes this protein to release and when it will be released is still unknown, but what we do know is that there are continual advances and changes in the understanding of the physiology of pregnancy, labour and birth.

In labour, there are a range of hormones interacting that include: Oxytocin, Endorphins, Prolactin, Vasopressin and Adrenaline.[10] Some of these hormones affect the parasympathetic nervous system and others the sympathetic nervous system. These two systems form the autonomic nervous system.

The autonomic nervous system stabilises the body's response to stress.[11] This part of the nervous system is responsible for control of the functions of the body that are involuntary, such as breathing, the heartbeat, and the process of digestion.

The autonomic nervous system is influenced by the birth hormones of oxytocin and adrenaline, both of which can be affected by the prenatal and postnatal yoga practices.

The Autonomic Nervous System

The autonomic nervous system is made up of the parasympathetic and sympathetic nervous systems. The parasympathetic nervous system is associated with calm and connection and is responsible for sensory and motor functions. The sympathetic nervous system is known as fight or flight, and is the survival system.

The vagus nerve interfaces with the parasympathetic nervous

system. In 2012, scientists at Boston University successfully showed that yoga positively affects the vagus nerve.[12] What they found was that because of the positive functioning of the nerve as a result of yoga practices, stress felt was reduced.

This understanding gives evidence of the benefit of a yoga practice during pregnancy as a way to reduce stress. Reduced stress allows for more efficient production of oxytocin, which in turn affects labour and breastfeeding.

The following table outlines the physiological processes through the body when the two systems are activated.

Parasympathetic	Sympathetic
Lowered blood pressure and heart rate	Increased heart rate and pumping volume
Increased circulation in the skin and mucous membranes	Elevated blood pressure
Lowered level of stress hormone	Increased blood circulation in the muscles
More effective digestion, nutritional intake and storage.	Extra fuel from release of glucose from the liver
	A higher level of stress hormone

By practising yoga through pregnancy and thus encouraging activation of the parasympathetic nervous system (while lowering stress), it allows better health for both mother and fetus. When the digestive system functions well, both mother and fetus receive more optimal nutrition.

The following table lists the birth hormones related to the parasympathetic nervous system and the sympathetic nervous system.

Parasympathetic	Sympathetic
Oxytocin	Vasopressin
Endorphins	Adrenaline family
Prolactin	

Oxytocin

Oxytocin is a key element in birth and breastfeeding and is responsible for some of the mother love feelings and bonding that can be present post birth. In-depth studies and information about the hormone is relatively new. That said, knowledge of love and theta, both of which can't be physically seen, have been well-known throughout the ages.

Oxytocin was discovered in 1906 by the English researcher, Sir Henry Dale. He discovered this hormone when he found that the uterus of a cat contracted with a substance from the pituitary gland. Oxytocin remains unchanged in every mammal and is commonly known as the love or the hug hormone. He named it oxytocin from the Greek words for "quick" and "birth".

The production of oxytocin is different to other hormones. Most hormones work with something known as a negative feedback loop.[13] What this means is that the body is regulated like how the temperature is controlled in a refrigerator. When the door is left open on a functioning fridge, the thermostat has to work harder to maintain the steady cold temperature. A similar process happens with most systems in the human body; there is in-built programming to maintain homeostasis. For example, when a person becomes too hot, a range of physiological processes such as sweating, dilation of the blood vessels close to the skin and the hairs near the skin lie flat. From these actions, the body usually returns to ideal temperature. Oxytocin production works in the opposite way to this and is on a positive feedback loop. Instead of trying to return to homeostasis, oxytocin production sees more oxytocin produced.

So in labour, when contractions start, oxytocin is released and this stimulates more contractions, which leads to more oxytocin being released and then more contractions. The cycle is self-limiting and continues until baby is born.

A similar process happens with breastfeeding. When a baby sucks their mothers breast, oxytocin is released which releases milk. With more sucking, more oxytocin and then more milk. Again, a self regulating cycle. When the baby has finished feeding, the oxytocin production ceases until the next feed. However, the opposite can also be true. If the production of oxytocin is interrupted by adrenaline or from other reasons, less oxytocin is produced until favourable conditions return. This can explain why a labour may stall and why a new mother may experience trouble with their milk supply if feeling anxious and stressed.

Becoming comfortable with being uncomfortable can be a way to relax into labour and make space for oxytocin production. We can't always control the environment externally but we can work at staying centred and non-reactive to both internal and external factors.

This parallels not only birth but also with parenthood. The practices of yoga teach people how to be in the moment: to work with what is happening each moment and discover ways to relax into what is happening in the now.

In birth and breastfeeding, maintaining practices that encourage oxytocin production, such as meditation and yoga, can be of great benefit.[14] These practices work on minimising adrenaline production and its possible effects.

Adrenaline

As humans, when we experience situations that are felt to be dangerous, the fight or flight reaction (activation of the sympathetic nervous system) happens with an adrenal reaction. When we are in pleasant and non-threatening situations, the rest and restore response (activation of the parasympathetic nervous system) is present, which is conducive to oxytocin production.

Each time a person reacts with an adrenal response, the body learns this reaction, and the next time, less of a stimulus is needed for a similar response. It has been found that hormones from the adrenal family are likely to restrain the proper functioning of the uterine muscles in birth.[15] Increases in adrenaline can also depress production of oxytocin, which in turn can slow labour and birth down.

Through pregnancy, reducing adrenal responses can also be an effective way to reduce stressful reactions through labour. The yoga and meditation practices are a way to do this.

Adrenaline is often seen as the enemy of a birthing room. Until the pushing stage, minimising factors that increase the production of adrenaline is beneficial. However, at pushing stage, adrenaline is necessary for efficient childbirth. Often women need that burst of adrenaline to have enough energy to push their baby out. What is becoming better understood is that there *is* a place for fear and adrenaline in the birthing room.[16] Rather than suggesting there is nothing to be afraid of, we can help prepare women to remain centred and in the moment.

So we must work with what is happening in the moment by minimising reactions of fear or denial, and also by preparing the mindset to birth in awareness.

The Uterus

The main muscles of labour are found in the uterus. By understanding the structure and function these muscles, we can build understanding of the physical and physiological process of labour. The uterus consists of a body and a cervix, and the cervix protrudes into the vagina.

The uterus is complex; it can grow from the size of a pear to the size of a watermelon[17] through pregnancy, and then back again post birth. Out of all of the body, oxytocin and adrenaline influence these muscles the most.

The uterus is composed of three layers. The inner layer is known as the endometrium, the middle layer is the myometrium and the outer layer is the perimetrium.[18]

For this book, we are mainly interested in the muscles of the middle layer, which are made up of three types of smooth muscles. Smooth muscles are involuntary in action and cannot be consciously controlled. For example, the flexing of the bicep in a voluntary muscle action. A person can decide to flex the muscle easily and on command. Intestinal muscle movement is an involuntary smooth muscle action; the intestine contracts without conscious direction. The muscles of the uterus work like the muscles of the intestines, from deep internal commands and knowing that is out of conscious control.

The smooth muscles that run lengthwise from the cervix, over the top of the uterus and back down to the cervix on the other side are the longitudinal muscles. They contract and shorten during labour, pulling up the cervix and pushing the baby down the birth canal. These muscles have two sources of nerve supply. The first is from the parasympathetic system and the second is from within the muscle itself. The longitudinal muscles work the best when the labouring woman is calm and unafraid. Grantley Dick-Reed, pioneer and inspirational author of 'Childbirth without Fear', extensively studied the uterus and discovered this to be so.

The second type form thick bundles that criss-cross and intertwine. The blood vessels running from the mother to the placenta pass through the openings of the loops in these figure eight shapes. The middle layer muscles prevent blood loss.

The third layer are circular. The nerve supply for the circular muscles come from fibres that are connected to stimulation from the sympathetic nervous system. When the circular muscles contract, the lower part of the uterus can become rigid. If this happens, then labour is slowed down or does not establish because the long and circular parts of the uterus are opposing each other.[19]

Parasympathetic	Sympathetic
Long muscles of uterus	Circular muscles of uterus
Stimulates the muscles of expulsion	Inhibit expulsion

For labour to progress and establish, it is more efficient to activate the calm and connection system. Yoga and breathing (the practices through these pages) positively activates and engages the parasympathetic nervous system.

The Neocortex

The neocortex is the 'new' part of the brain. It's related to intellectual activities and is responsible for language. It is stimulated when we engage in intellectual activity and when we feel we are being observed. The neocortex is behind why much of the information gathered, read and intellectualised about birth in the preparation time can be forgotten and unable to be accessed in labour.

In birth, the neocortex needs to be at rest so that the pituitary gland and the hypothalamus (which release oxytocin and are in charge of vital functions such as giving birth) can fully function.

Intellectual stimulation and rational language stimulates the neocortex, as do bright lights and a feeling of being watched. Michel Odent, a leading French obstetrician, often writes about the need of humans in birth to be protected from the stimulation of the neocortex.[20]

Part of what we teach in prenatal yoga classes are practices to reduce the influence of the neocortex. Repeating the asana, breathing practices and building awareness helps women achieve this when they move into labour. Instead of having to think about what to do, after repeated practice, the body remembers and moves from a place of knowing rather than thinking. People who struggle to stay rational and in control reactivate the neocortex, which can work against the functioning of labour.

The function of the brain shifts through pregnancy and birth. The left side of the brain is largely responsible for planning, thinking, strategising, linear thought; the masculine. The right side of the brain is more for creativity, symbols, images, art; the feminine.

In regular day-to-day life, both sides are active and cross over. Once labour is established, the left side of the brain and its functions shut down, leaving the labouring woman in her right hemisphere, that of non-linear thought. Rational thought makes way for visualisations, affirmations, art and flowing movement – which are all still accessible. The brain also treats obscenities differently to other words, which is why a woman deep in established labour may start swearing!

Relaxin

Relaxin is a hormone produced in both pregnant and non-pregnant women. In non-pregnant women and those in the early stages of pregnancy it is produced by the corpus luteum, which is a yellow mass left behind in the ovaries following ovulation.[21]

The amount of relaxin builds through the pregnancy. In the second trimester, the placenta and the lining of the uterus take over the production. Production ceases with delivery of the placenta and resumes with the recommencement of the menstrual cycle. Relaxin stays in the body for up to six months post birth and in some cases even longer.

The levels of relaxin are higher in second and subsequent pregnancies and in women carrying more than one baby. The effects of this increased relaxin on the body during pregnancy are most significant in the collagen part of the connective tissue.[22] There is an increase in elasticity yet decreased strength, and joint stability is the most affected.[23] Due to this, relaxin has a significant effect on the physical practice of yoga.

There are a high number of relaxin receptors located in the pelvis and this contributes to flexibility. The pelvic joints are allowed a greater range of movement as a result of the increased elasticity. Depending on the birth position, the pelvic outlet may increase by about 30 per cent during delivery.[24]

However, the hormone relaxin can't only be released in the pelvic joints, so there is the risk of overstretching other parts of the body. Relaxin can cause instability and abnormal motion of the sacroiliac joint, pubic symphysis and other joints, that can cause considerable pain.

It is these areas that particular care needs to be taken when teaching or practising prenatal yoga. In a prenatal class, it is necessary to regulate the depth of asana and also the length of time people are in asanas. For a pregnant woman in a general class, asanas such as lunges can greatly affect these areas if held for too long or too deeply. At the time of the class the effects are generally not noticed; it is usually post practice that the impact is felt. Thus, it can be difficult for a pregnant woman to know if she is stretching too deeply until some damage is already done. It is useful to discuss this with pregnant students and for them to be aware of possible complications from overstretching.

To greatly reduce the risk of ligamental damage, it is recommended that people's yoga practice does not go much deeper than their range of movement and flexibility pre-pregnancy.

Relaxin also affects muscles. The muscles of the abdomen undergo the greatest change through pregnancy as they stretch to allow the uterus to grow. The pelvic floor muscles also endure increasing pressure during pregnancy and are stretched (and may even tear) during birth.

Although production of relaxin ceases on delivery of the placenta, connective tissue changes that have occurred will continue until new tissue has been re-formed without relaxin. The ligaments should return to their pre-pregnancy state once the effects of relaxin have left the body. Breastfeeding women may find increased joint laxity continues until feeding stops. This is because prolactin's suppressive effects on oestrogen production contributes to lack of strength and stiffness in connective tissue, which may in turn prolong joint instability.

Chapter FIVE

The Pelvic Floor

Through pregnancy and birth, the main damage to the pelvic floor is from the pressure resulting from increased weight on the sling of muscles over the nine months of pregnancy. Understanding the structure of the pelvic floor builds awareness of what can be done to maintain these muscles.

The core, diaphragm and the pelvic floor are all interconnected and work together to stabilise and control through the body. Breath and posture affect and are effected by these groups of muscles. Learning how to engage and relax through the pelvic floor is useful for birth, as these muscles need to be relaxed in the pushing stage.

The Anatomy of the Pelvic Floor

The pelvic floor muscles are responsible for supporting the pelvic organs, for sexual function, and supporting women through pregnancy and birth. The muscles of the pelvic floor also work with the diaphragm and abdominal and back muscles to stabilise and support the spine and control pressure in the abdomen.

There are three layers of pelvic floor muscles.[25] The first layer of the pelvic floor attaches the tip of the tail bone to the pubic symphysis with a figure eight shape. There is a left and right side and it is the most superficial layer. This layer is known as the superficial perineal pouch. The second layer and middle layer of the pelvic floor is transverse and crosses perineum. It is known as the urogenital diaphragm. The deepest layer is known as the pelvic diaphragm.

Anatomy of the Pelvic Floor

1st layer	2nd layer	Deepest layer
Superficial Transverse Perineal	Deep Transverse Perineal	Levator Ani (Pubococcygeus-pubovaginalis, puborectalis, and Iliococcygeus)
Bulbocavernosus	Sphincter urethrovaginalis	Coccygeus
Ischiocavernosus	Compressor Urethra	
External Anal Sphincter	External Urethral Sphincter	

The Core

The core muscles stabilise the body. These deep abdominal muscles affect and are affected by both the pelvic floor and the diaphragm as it engages with each breath.

The abdominal muscles are layered. From the most superficial, they are: rectus abdominus, external obliques, internal obliques and the deepest layer: the transverse abdominus.[26]

The rectus abdominus muscles and transverse abdominus are the two sets of muscles that we focus on in yoga during pregnancy and birth. The rectus abdominus muscles need to soften and the deep transverse abdominus muscles need to engage.

The obliques are responsible for twisting movements and these movements are minimised during pregnancy.

Dysfunction of the transverse abdominus muscles is common during pregnancy and birth. Often people let their core strength release completely and use their more superficial abdominal muscles or their back muscles to do the work. This can lead to imbalances and back pain. Or they use the superficial rectus abdominus muscles, and this can lead to separation.

In a cesarean birth, the abdominal muscles themselves are not actually cut. The fascia surrounding each layer is cut, which gives the obstetrician space to move the muscles around to be able to birth the baby.

Rectus Abdominus

The outermost layer of the abdominals are the rectus abdominus muscles; often referred to as the abs. These are the muscles that can separate through pregnancy and post birth, and the images below illustrate what happens to these muscles when that happens.

With abdominal separation, women can suffer from a reduced core strength and pelvic floor instability.

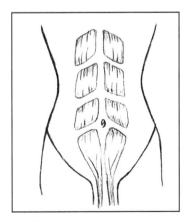

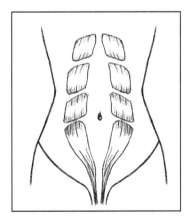

Diagram 1: approximate representation of rectus abdominus

Diagram 2: approximate representation of abdominal separation

Often the consequence of this is lower back pain.

Transverse Abdominus

The transverse abdominus muscles are the deepest set of core muscles, located under the rectus abdominus and the internal and external obliques.

Transverse abdominus are the body's major expulsion muscles, so building and maintaining strength through here can greatly assist the pushing phase of labour.

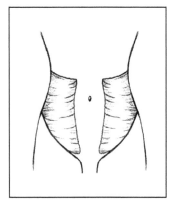

Diagram 1: approximate representation of the transverse abdominus

A transverse abdominus test

To test if these transverse abdominus muscles are activating and engaging, lie on your back as if preparing for bridge and lift through one heel, with the toes pressing into the mat. It is a subtle movement as the muscles are so deep.

If teaching, ensure participants do not press up through their bellies and engage the rectus abdominus muscles as they are lifting their heels. If these muscles are activating there is a feeling of deep engagement, while the more superficial muscles are soft.

If no activation is felt, start slowly with gentle strengthening and re-building exercises. Heel raises, with awareness, are the starting point of engagement and strengthening. Follow this with full feet lifts once activation is noticeable. Ensure at all times that the superficial muscles are at rest.

Women suffering major abdominal separation need to work on this with a physiotherapist before being able to fully engage in these exercises.

Posture, Core and the Pelvic Floor

Posture influences the pelvic floor muscles and so if there is an issue with the pelvic floor muscles, the support of the spine can be compromised. During pregnancy, core strength is already compromised due to the growing uterus, so the back body is more heavily relied upon for support and stability. Building awareness of the spine, both in sitting and standing positions, along with releasing the surrounding muscles through the asana practice, can lead to a stronger and more stable posture.

From this stable posture, awareness and improved function of the pelvic floor is possible. If practising pelvic floor muscle exercises in the car at traffic lights, be aware of posture as the seat of most cars encourages a slumped sitting position.

The following illustrations depict the three common ways people stand.

Ideal Posture

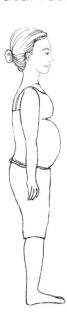

The head is straight, with the chin tucked in slightly. Shoulders are in line without rolling forward, and the natural curves of the spine are present without being exaggerated. During pregnancy, ideal posture is often compromised and there is often a more pronounced lordosis (which is pronounced inward curve of the spine) through the lower back. The added weight through the breasts and abdominal region can result in forward movement through the upper back.

Computer work and much desk sitting can contribute to poor posture. When repeatedly done, it can lead to a shift in the shape of the skeleton and the function of the muscles of the region.

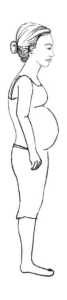

Forward head and sway back (lordosis)

The curve through the lower back is exaggerated. The shoulders generally sit back and the head thrusts forward. The stomach pushes further forward and creates more instability through the core.

In pregnancy, the core is already compromised. The breath may be restricted, as well as the pelvic floor function, due to a tilt in the pelvis.

As ideal posture does rely on core strength, sometimes there may be a compromise with core strength and back posture. Women who do too much core strengthening can compromise the health and stability of their core muscles, and this can lead to a condition through either pregnancy or postpartum known as *abdominal separation*.

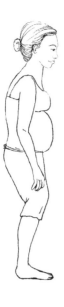

Forward head and flat back (kyphosis)

The curve through the upper back increases and the shoulders roll forward, increasing pressure on the head and neck. The lower back starts to flatten, which results in distortion with the tilt of the pelvis.

An extreme example of this posture is a hunched over person with a hump back. The lungs and thus breath becomes restricted in this posture. The pelvic floor may become compromised.

The Breath, the Core and the Pelvic Floor

When you breathe in, the diaphragm contracts and moves down towards the abdomen. The diaphragm relaxes and moves upward on the exhalation. Breathing by fully engaging the diaphragm affects the pelvic floor because when you breathe in deeply during diaphragmatic breathing, the pressure inside the abdomen is increased. So the pelvic floor muscles need to contract even more strongly to maintain your continence. From here, the transverse abdominus muscles engage effectively with each exhalation.

When women 'chest breathe' and do not use their diaphragm fully, the core and pelvic floor do not engage properly with each breath. By changing the depth of a breath, the pelvic floor muscles can be engaged while breathing, thus becoming more toned and active.

When women use their diaphragm fully and engage their pelvic floor, they can also increase the strength and efficiency of their core muscles. One way this can be beneficial during pregnancy and post-partum is a movement known as the pelvic brace—which is outlined later in this chapter.

The pelvic floor muscles can be overly tight or overly loose and this depends on a range of conditioning. The table below gives a way to visualise the health of a muscle based on its range of motion. A tight muscle is a weak muscle... a slack muscle is a weak muscle... and neither can move very much.

Tight and weak muscles	Clenched fist that can't open
Long and weak muscles	Open hand that can't clench

The following table outlines the signs of overly tight pelvic floor muscles and overly loose pelvic floor muscles.

Signs of an overly tight (hypertonic) pelvic floor	Signs of a lax (hypotonic) pelvic floor
Urge incontinence or the constant need to urinate	Stress incontinence
The whole body is overly tight	Overweight
Tightness in the jaw, neck, shoulders	Sedentary
Pelvis is retroverted/posterior tilted/tucked (flat back)	Pelvis is more anteriorly tilted (lordosis)
Painful intercourse, vulva pain	Hysterectomy
Sedentary, while seated has rounded lumbar	Menopause
Digestive issues, ie constipation, irritable bowel syndrome, cystitis	Multiple births
Chest breather	Lack of sensation during intercourse
Traumatic or prolonged births (births that require a lot of pushing, episiotomy, and/or forceps	Prolapse of pelvic organs
Any experience that was intrusive (including surgery) that caused emotional or physical scarring	Experience of passing air through the vagina during sex or inversions
	Breath may be present in the belly but much more towards the front of the body

Pelvic floor muscles can become hyper-tense when they are without full awareness of which muscles are being engaged. Alternatively, the gluteal muscles or the hamstrings may be engaged and the pelvic floor muscles become slack. There are different reasons for this. So if women are unsure of what's happening, they can visit a women's physiotherapist and discover the functioning of their pelvic floor, with real time ultrasound.

Pelvic Floor Exercises

Pelvic floor exercises can make up an important part of a prenatal and postpartum yoga practice. Practised correctly they can positively influence the health of the pelvic floor muscles.

There are two types of pelvic floor exercises and they work the quick- and slow-release fibres of the muscles. Both are important to learn and practise.

When teaching these exercises, it can be useful to briefly explain the structure of the pelvic floor and the surrounding muscles before starting the exercises, so women can locate the muscles and have an understanding of what muscles they need to engage.

In general classes, pregnant women can practise the pelvic floor exercises seated or standing if there is an asana or sequence that is contraindicated for them.

Key Points to Remember

The following are key points to remember when practising the pelvic floor exercises.

- ◎ Exhale while lifting and ensure you do not push down when breath releases
- ◎ Keep the forehead and jaw relaxed

- ◉ Avoid any bend at the waist
- ◉ Be aware of keeping the buttocks relaxed and not engaged throughout the exercises.

Slow Release

- ◉ Inhale with a full belly breath;
- ◉ On the exhalation, draw the pelvic floor muscles together from the left and right and engage around the front area;
- ◉ Lift up inside;
- ◉ Hold for a few seconds while continuing to breathe;
- ◉ Release and lower with control.

This can be repeated 10 times. If people are unable to do 10, then as many as possible.

Quick Release

- ◉ Tighten and lift pelvic floor muscles as high as possible in one quick contraction;
- ◉ Release immediately.

This can be repeated 10 times. If people are unable to do 10, then as many as possible.

The Pelvic Brace

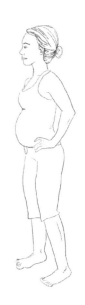

The pelvic brace is a way to support posture and is a term I picked up from Isa Herrera, a pelvic floor expert. It can be the difference between pelvic pain during pregnancy or postpartum and relief. The pelvic brace is low level engagement of the pelvic floor, with the transverse abdominals engaged. In yoga, it is the simultaneous and gentle engagement of the Mula and Uddiyana Bandhas.

The Bandhas

Pelvic floor engagement is called Mula Bandha and the transverse abdominus is a part of Uddiyana Bandha.

If you are teaching a class full of experienced yoga students, it can be beneficial to discuss the bandhas and how they relate to pregnancy, birth and post-birth recovery from an anatomical perspective.

In Sanskrit, mula means root, and thus Mula Bandha is *the root lock*. To find it, sit, stand, or even be in an asana, contract the muscles at the bottom of the pelvic floor, behind the cervix.

In Sanskrit, uddiyana means to fly up, or to rise up. This 'flying up lock' is thus all about your insides flying upwards, intangibly meaning your energy, tangibly meaning your diaphragm, stomach, and abdominal organs. Full Uddiyana Bandha is contraindicated for pregnant women as this involves strong abdominal movements and breath retention.

Chapter SIX

Teaching Prenatal Yoga

When teaching pregnant women yoga, practise and explore different levels of intensity on yourself. Explore yourself, and you will be more open to give others the space to explore deeply within. How do you cope? Where does your mind go? If there is an asana that causes you extreme discomfort, do you try to avoid that one?

Exploring these questions within can develop insight into what students may be going through. Observing yourself in your practice opens the way for you to observe others. As complex as we all think we are, in many ways we are very similar.

When you teach, teach from your heart. Find your voice. With the clarity and space you cultivate, you can share it with your students. Allow your journey and you will be able to hold space to allow theirs. Invite your students to notice their internal chatter whenever a position causes them discomfort. Explore their responses to discomfort. Have them build awareness of how they may resist or embrace the sensations.

If any discomfort is felt—beyond a normal stretching sensation—guide students to reduce intensity. If they are concerned about pains or unusual sensations then they need to speak to their obstetrician, doctor or midwife. As a prenatal yoga teacher, you are not a medical practitioner and cannot diagnose or give medical advice.

When teaching women through their pregnancy, either in a specific prenatal yoga class or by modifying an asana practice, listen to the individual and respond from your heart space. Often the relationships women have through pregnancy and birth are more important than the outcomes they achieve. There is transformation and growth each moment throughout pregnancy. The interactions you have with your pregnant students can be as powerful for them as it is for you, their yoga teacher.

Pregnancy can stir up a range of emotions and so women experience fluctuations throughout their pregnancy. Not all pregnancies are planned or are welcome surprises, and it can take time to process. Be sensitive to emotions and let them flow in class. Some women may cry during the practice and that could be the release they need. Be careful not to interrupt someone's process and be sensitive to their needs.

Your Voice

When yoga is taught from the heart, students can hear it through their ears and through their bodies. It is the difference between yoga and doing gymnastics. When I first started teaching yoga, I had returned to Sydney from India. The owners of the studio who hired me were so supportive and loving. Each Sunday morning, one of the owners would turn up to the class and support me through his presence, his eyes and his feedback. Knowing that I didn't have to try to be right or perfect, rather authentic and teach from my heart, allowed the students to practise from that space as well.

When students feel that space in a prenatal yoga class, they can also take it with them through their pregnancy and birth. We are not preparing students to try to get their birth right, but rather to be present and aware in their own space which will be different to everyone else's. Speak from your experience and authentic self. When you have accessed that voice you can hold the space for the students to explore.

Chapter SEVEN

Prenatal Yoga Contraindications

Contraindications

There are a range of common issues, signs and symptoms that women can have in pregnancy. They can appear suddenly and unexpectedly. As a prenatal yoga teacher, check in with students each time you see them. If there is new information, you need to be aware of this before beginning the practice. If any conditions are presented that you are not familiar with, check with the student that she has had approval from her caregiver / medical practitioner to practise yoga.

If you are using this book for your own pregnancy yoga practice, regularly check the contraindications and conditions as you progress through pregnancy. With care, knowledge and awareness, everyone can continue with a yoga practice through pregnancy by making the right adjustments and changes.

The asanas are not meant as a replacement of any treatment that other health professionals may have given. These guidelines are related to yoga, what to include or leave out of a practice, and how to modify a practice. It is outside the scope of practice for a yoga teacher to give any kind of medical advice.

If symptoms worsen after practising an asana, women need to discuss the issue with a caregiver for advice/diagnosis before continuing the yoga practice.

Conditions and Adjustments

Condition	Recommendations
Varicose veins	Avoid Squats
	Practise Legs up Wall with a prop to avoid full supine position
Pubic Symphysis	Avoid one-footed asana
	Be careful of width in open-legged asana
	Gomukasana may help
	Virasana rather than cross-legged for seated meditations
High blood pressure	Deep relaxation. May be beneficial to do yoga nidra/relaxations daily
	Avoid Forward Bends
	Modify any poses where hands are held above the head
Low blood pressure	Avoid head below shoulders
	Avoid Down Dog
	If dizzy, take rest
Nausea	May need a small snack through the practice

Condition	Recommendations
Nausea (continued)	Careful not to have too much flowing movement if this increases the nausea
Carpal Tunnel Syndrome	Keep wrists neutral – use a fist, making sure wrist is in alignment with any positions on hands and knees
Constipation	Practise Virasana
	Squats
	A change in diet may be beneficial
Heartburn	Sitting in Virasana while eating (and for 15 minutes after) can aid digestion
Fluid retention	Wrist and ankle circling
	Legs up Wall with a fusion to avoid full supine
Back Pain	This is a common symptom in pregnancy and often this can't be removed, rather relieved. Most of the asana will work with the spine and open up the body.
	Check posture
	Diaphramatic breathing
	Child's pose to take weight off spine
	Neck and shoulder exercises for upper back tension
	Avoid extending the spine backward until after birth when back strengthens.

Condition	Recommendations
Cramping in legs	Practise Down Dog
	Practise Janur Sirsasana
	Sit in Virasana
	Check hydration. Cramping can be caused by dehydration.
Haemorroids	Avoid Squats
Breech baby	Avoid Squats after 35 weeks
	Practise supported bridge and also look into optimal foetal positioning.
	Spinning babies is a great resource that you can offer students to go and explore **www.spinningbabies.com**
Placenta Previa	Avoid full squatting
	Lessen the distance between legs for Warrior 2 and modify Butterfly by taking the feet further away from the body and propping hips on a bolster.
Posterior baby	Hands and knees hip rotations
	Check seated posture – there's evidence that slumping in a chair can encourage posterior turn.
	Again, spinning babies can be a good resource to work with optimal foetal positioning. **www.spinningbabies.com**
Excess amniotic fluid	Practise Down Dog

The following conditions can occur in pregnancy and so if a student lets you know she has any of the below, check with her that she has discussed practising yoga with her caregiver.

Yoga can be beneficial for these conditions, but as a yoga teacher you are not trained to diagnose or know the severity of any condition. It is each person's responsibility to have discussed their yoga practice with their doctor or midwife before continuing with asana practice.

Diabetes
Pre-eclampsia
High blood pressure
Low blood pressure
Severe anaemia

High Risk Factors

The following are signs and symptoms of high risk factors of pregnancy and conditions that need caregiver approval to practise prenatal yoga. If a student presents with the below conditions and has not had approval from her doctor or midwife to practice yoga, advise them they will need this before continuing with yoga asana.

Asanas to avoid

Some asanas need to be avoided during pregnancy. As a general rule, there should never be deep compression, twisting or extreme stretching of the abdomen. Inversions or jumping could compromise the placenta and should be avoided.

Avoid full supine, flat back lying after the first trimester. During pregnancy, also avoid breath retention.

The following table goes into more detail for all pregnant students.

Asana	Reason to avoid
Abdominal twists and any deep twisting	Decreases blood circulation. Can compress the uterus and also place unnecessary pressure on the placenta.
Inversions	Balance can be an issue but the main risk with inversions, especially for the experienced practitioner, are that they can also rupture the placenta.
Extreme back bends	Can overstretch the abdominals and also compress the uterus.
Prone positions (eg. Cobra, Up dog)	Compresses the uterus and puts a lot of pressure on both the fetus and placenta.
Supine postures with flat back	Compresses the vena cava and can also aggravate lower back pain, heartburn, and elevate blood pressure
Jumping	Risk of rupturing the placenta and puts unnecessary pressure on the pelvic floor
Standing forward folds with head completely down	Folding forward can compress blood vessels and nerves that connect to your uterus. Separating the legs to minimise compression. Do not go too deeply and be careful not to compress the belly.

Asana	Reason to avoid
Overstretching	Can over-loosen the ligaments and create instability through the body. The main area of concern is the pubic symphysis, which if overstretched can be painful and lead to pelvic instability that can continue post birth.
Child's pose with legs together	Compression of belly and uterus.
Breath retention	May restrict oxygen to the fetus and can cause a blackout if this was to happen, as an internal survival mechanism triggers to ensure the woman keeps breathing.
Strong abdominal poses	Overly strong obliques can pull the abdominal muscles apart, causing diastasis recti.

Chapter EIGHT

Asanas

The Asanas

The asanas are the postures adopted in the yoga practice and in this book they are categorised according to type of position. Included categories are: kneeling, hands and knees, squats, standing, arms and shoulders, seated, side lying, hips, back-bending and relaxation.

The following can give ideas of what asana can be used as a substitute in a general yoga practice or they can be used to plan a full prenatal yoga practice. There are some suggested sequences in the appendix of the book.

Unless otherwise indicated, hold each asana for between five and ten breaths. Ensure that both sides of the body are balanced.

The asanas included are generally safe for pregnancy. Refer to the list of contraindications for specific conditions. Before starting a prenatal yoga practice, check with a medical provider.

Kneeling

The kneeling series incorporates stretching and stamina building options for physical and emotional release. The kneeling asanas can be practised at the beginning or end of the session and also interwoven through the practice.

The kneeling position is an alternative seated position for anyone unable to sit cross-legged. The pubic symphysis is stable in this position and is thus ideal for women suffering from pubic symphysis pain through pregnancy. In this position, the spine can be lengthened for meditation.

Instead of pressing the buttocks into the heels in the positions, they can be modified by lifting hips off the feet altogether, to a high kneeling position. Alternatively, place a bolster, cushion or folded blanket on the calves to prop up and support the hips.

Thunderbolt

vajrasana

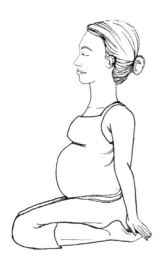

Benefits

Sitting in this posture can relieve sciatic pain. Ideal for people suffering from constipation or who are having trouble digesting. An alternative for people who are unable to sit cross-legged.

How to

Flex the knees with the shins on the mat and press hips onto or between the heels. Hands rest on feet as illustrated, or on the knees, with the fingers pointing away from the body and the palms facing down. If there is pain in the knees, place a bolster on the back of the shins to support the hips.

Lions Breath in Thunderbolt
simhasana

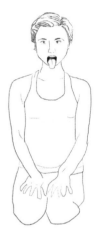

Benefits

Relieves tension through the face and neck. Encourages people to make noise and funny faces without worrying what others may think—which can be great preparation for labour.

How to

From a kneeling position, place hands on knees with the fingers opened, just as a feline may open their paws. Start with a deep inhalation through the nose and open the mouth wide and stretch the tongue out. Exhale slowly through the mouth, with the eyes open wide and the muscles on the front of your throat contracted, making a haaaaaaaaa sound. Close the mouth at the end of the exhalation to inhale through the nose. Repeat as many times as desired.

Toe Tuck

Benefits

The asana releases the planta fascia, which can be painful at the time, but intimately deeply nourishing. Yet it can be particularly challenging for women who wear heeled shoes. This is a 'stay focused and stay centred' asana, and one that is valuable as preparation for contractions and practising ways of coping with body intensity.

How to

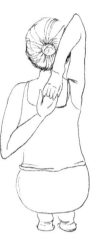

From a kneeling position, tuck the toes under so they are stretching back. Try to be on the balls of the feet and lean into the heels. Keep the knees on the mat. If sitting back on the heels is too strong, move into a kneeling position to relieve pressure on the toe joints, returning to the deep position when able. Hands can be resting on the knees, or to intensify, clasp hands behind the back as illustrated.

Hands and Knees

The asana practised on hands and knees are either strengthening, releasing or a combination of both. They are useful as a preparation for labour as women often spend quite a lot of their labour on their hands and knees. There are many old stories around of women who scrubbed the floors on their hands and knees who were naturally optimising their fetal position and preparing their bodies for birth.

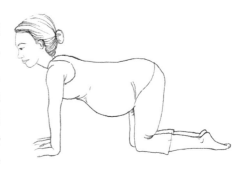

With any of the positions where wrist pain or carpel tunnel syndrome is present while the wrist is extended, it is necessary to neutralise the wrists. This can be done by making fists with both hands and pressing into the end of the fingers, with thumbs facing forward. Another option is to take all pressure off the wrist joints and come onto the forearms by bending at the elbows, with palms facing down.

If there is abdominal separation, ensure the abdomen does not fully drop on any of the hands/knees positions as this adds too much pressure to the already-weakened core and lower back. Transverse abdominal and pelvic floor activation can support the core from the hands and knees positions. (See page 44 for the pelvic brace instructions).

Hands and Knees Posture

How to

From a kneeling position, open knees to hip width distance apart. On an exhalation, place palms of the hands on the mat, shoulder width distance apart, with wrists under the shoulders. Engage the palms and press all knuckles into the mat, with the middle fingers pointing forward.

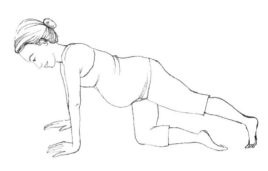

Options

Alternate flexion and extension of the wrists. From the hands and knees position, extend one wrist while keeping the other wrist in flexion and then alternate from side to side. The hands can move with quick paddling movements or be held longer (approximately 30 seconds on each side).

Deep circling through the hips and shoulders. From the hands and knees position, take the knees out to either side of the mat and move them back approximately ten centimetres. On an exhalation, circle the hips back towards the heels as deeply as is comfortable.

On an inhalation, circle the body forward and around. Moving in a rhythm with breath is a free circular motion, as quickly or slowly as desired. After ten breaths, change direction of the circling for ten more breaths. To release, return to neutral.

Hands-and-Knees Calf Stretch

Benefits

Lengthens through the calves. Can be relieving if suffering from cramping through the legs.

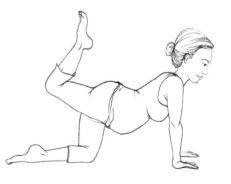

How to

From the hands and knees position,

inhale to lift the right leg, extend the leg and press the ball of the right foot into the mat while extending through the toes. Draw the heel towards the mat and keep the neck neutral and the crown of the head reaching forwards. This can be a static hold or the heel can pump forwards and backwards.

To release, on an inhalation, lift the right foot and flex through the right knee. Return to neutral on the exhalation. Repeat on the left side.

Options

The calf stretch can also be practised standing against a wall (see p.82).

Hands-and-Knees Bent Knee Lift and Hip Opener

Benefits

Releases and stretches through the hips and hip flexors. Gentle abdominal strengthening and increases balance.

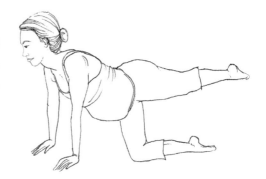

How to

From the hands and knees position, on an inhalation flex through the knee of the right leg and lift the leg, pointing the toes towards the ceiling. On each exhalation, open through the front of the thigh and take the toes a little higher. Keep spine neutral and hold for 5 breaths. Release the knee to the mat on an exhalation. Repeat on the left side.

Options

Hip opening circles. With the right knee flexed and raised, circle through the hips in a clockwise direction, and then an anti-clockwise position for deep opening through the hips. Use the breath to work with the circular movements. Inhale to circle up and exhale for the movement back.

Leg Extension

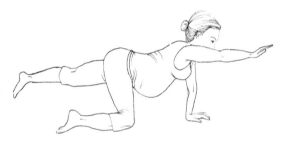

Benefits

Encourages core strength and balance. Encourages awareness of breath when trying to hold balance.

How to

From the hands and knees position, find a point and focus the gaze. On an inhalation raise and extend the right leg, with toes pointed directly behind. Hold the balance while maintaining a steady flow of breath. On an exhalation lower knee to mat to release. Repeat on the left side.

Leg Extension with Optional Arm Extension

Benefits

This position encourages core strength and balance. Women in the position work with their breath to stabilise, an important practice for labour and birth preparation.

How to

From the leg extension position with the right leg, on an inhalation raise and extend the left arm, with palm facing the mat. Lengthen through the right leg and left arm for 5 breaths.

To release, place the hand and knee on the mat with an exhalation. Repeat with the left leg and right arm. Take to a 45 degree angle for an intercostal stretch.

To protect and support the lower back, engage the transverse abdominus muscles and pelvic floor muscles in the pelvic brace. (See page 44).

Optional: Additional core strengthening

Draw the elbow and bent knee in towards each other on an exhalation and extend on an inhalation.

Repeat 5 times on each side for abdominal strengthening.

Cat/Cow

marjarayasana/bitilasana

Benefits

Stretches and strengthens the spine and the neck. Stretches through the hips, abdomen and back.

Practise this asana through contractions to soften the pelvis and encourage movement of the fetus towards the birth canal (more likely in the earlier contractions before they get too intense).

An active position without high intensity, allowing great movement through the spine and pelvis.

Practising these asana can encourage the movement of a posterior baby. When people are on all fours, the back of the baby's head swings to the front of the belly.

How to

˜ Cat ˜

From the hands and knees position, round the spine up towards the ceiling on the exhalation and imagine pulling the belly button up towards the spine.

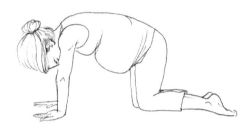

˜ Cow ˜

On the inhalation, draw the shoulder blades in towards each other and lift through the head while releasing through the lower back.

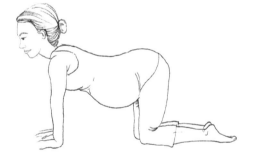

Keep spine neutral on the inhalation if there is instability through the sacroiliac joint, abdominal separation, limited/no core support or pronounced lordosis in the lower back. In the later stages of pregnancy stay neutral because the pressure from the downward movement can strain the back muscles and ligaments.

Down Dog
adho mukha svanasana

Benefits

A stretching and strengthening asana for both the upper and lower body.

Through the legs there is lengthening of the hamstrings and opening through the upper back.

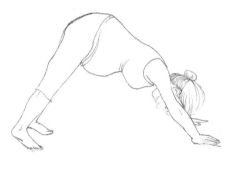

Boosts circulation and strengthens bone density, which can often be compromised during pregnancy.

How to

From the hands and knees position, on an exhalation tuck toes, lift knees off the mat, extend the legs and press the floor away with the hands to draw the pelvis upwards. The knees can remain bent and the heels can be lifted off the mat to flatten through the back.

Hold for 1 to 5 breaths and release on an inhalation by bringing knees back onto the mat.

Modify

The modified wall position is an option (p. 81).

Practice tips

Down Dog is a type of inversion where the head is below the heart. From 30 weeks, it should not be held for longer than 30 seconds. There is no firm evidence to show that baby can flip from optimal head down position to breech in this inversion. Once a fetus is engaged, it will not dis-engage. However, from week 36, many women prefer to stay upright as it can feel uncomfortable with the positioning of the fetus.

Gate Pose

parighasana

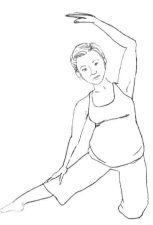

Benefits

Stretches the intercostal muscles and opens the side body. Releases tension through the neck and shoulders.

How to

From a kneeling position, extend the right leg out to the side while keeping the right heel inline with the left knee. Keep the left thigh in a vertical line as support and activate the right leg. The right toes can point forward as illustrated or out to the side.

On an inhalation raise the left arm and place the right hand along the right leg. On an exhalation reach the left fingertips, with palm facing down, towards the right side of the body. Hold for 5 breaths.

To release, raise arms on an inhalation and on the exhalation release hands and bring the right knee back to the kneeling position. Repeat with the left leg.

Child's Pose
balasana

Benefits

Stretches the ankles, thighs, hips and knees and releases back and neck tension. A calming posture that relieves stress and fatigue.

Being in this position can activate the parasympathetic nervous system and so can be a calming position to be in before sleep. As a preparation for birth, this is an ideal position to take rest between contractions, which is as important for birth as the contractions themselves.

How to

From hands and knees position, widen knees to either side of the mat and draw the big toes towards each other to touch if possible. On an exhalation, draw hips back towards the heels and slide hands out towards the front of the mat. Lengthen through the arms on the inhalation and further release hips on the exhalation.

Keep hips high in the air if there seems to be any pressure through the abdomen; this is more common during the later stages of pregnancy.

If it is not comfortable extending the arms out in front, create a cushion with the hands on top of each other for the forehead to rest on.

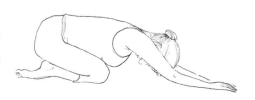

Revolved Child's Pose

parsva balasana

Benefits

Releases shoulder, chest, upper
back and neck tension.

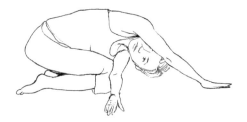

How to

From hands and knees position,
take knees to either side of the
mat and have big toes touching, if comfortable. Keep hips as raised as
necessary. On an inhalation, raise up the right arm and on the exhalation slide the right arm underneath the left shoulder. The right shoulder comes onto the mat while resting head and neck down.

Place a bolster underneath the head to keep a more upright position if needed. To release, press into the left hand to support and take
the right arm out, reaching the right fingertips up towards the ceiling.
Exhale the right hand back to the mat. Repeat with the left arm.

Squats

Squats can be powerful asana for pregnancy and birth preparation and there are a range of squats that can be practised during a class. They strengthen, release, and can help build awareness of internal resistance as a pain-coping practice. Squats are another option for the 'stay focused and stay centred' practice. By having women hold static squats for about a minute—to work with the length of a typical contraction—they can be an effective way of exploring any resistance to body sensations.

By adding movement to the arms or legs to make the squat dynamic, we can explore how movement can work as a distraction while experiencing strong sensations.

Dynamic squats can also be strengthening and warming.

I recently learned from a Canadian Doula that in some traditional groups in Canada, at pushing stage, the women do not open their knees wider than a fist width's distance (so there is no internal rotation of the femur bones) in birth to allow the pelvis full expansion and to protect the perineum.

You can experiment with your own body by palpating (touching) your sitting bones and feel the difference to the pelvis when you open the knees out versus pressing the knees together with a fist between the knees. I also heard from a midwife that they observed more tearing and pressure on the perineum with very wide upright squatting positions in the pushing stage.

If women do not feel comfortable in squats, it is important for them to listen to their bodies and decide to participate or not. Squats should also be avoided with the following conditions:

- Pubic symphysis
- An incompetent cervix or if there is premature dilation of the cervix

- ◎ Knee issues
- ◎ Haemorrhoids
- ◎ Varicose veins

Deep Squat
malasana

Benefits

Releases through the hips and groin, making it an ideal pose for birth preparation. Stretches through the hamstrings, ankles, back and neck. Strengthens through the body and mind.

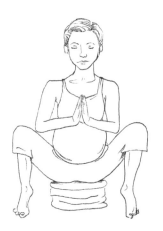

How to

From standing, step feet to either side of the mat and point toes out to a 45 degree angle, keeping the heels on the mat. Bend the knees to lower into a squat. Place elbows on the inside of the knees as illustrated by leaning forward slightly and pressing hands together into a prayer position. Hands can stay resting on the knees or on the back of a chair if keeping balance is challenging and it is difficult to bring the hands into prayer. Feet can be flat on the floor or on the toes as illustrated and use a folded blanket under the heels to support if needed.

To modify, sit on a towel or bolster, with the option to also lean against the wall if there is pain in the knees.

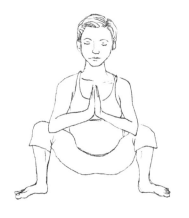

Unsupported deep squat

Strengthening Squat

jiva balasana

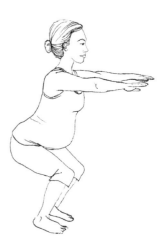

Benefits

Strengthens through the thigh muscles and increases pelvic floor muscle strength. Builds resistance through the arms.

How to

From a standing position, step feet parallel and hip width apart, but if balance is challenged the feet can be wider than parallel. Extend both arms forward with palms facing down and parallel to the mat. On an exhalation, flex through the knees, positioning the hips so they are not lower than the knees. To stabilise, softly engage the pelvic floor perineal region when holding the position. Hold for a minute and release on an exhale, engaging the pelvic floor gently to extend through the knees, releasing hands to the sides of the body.

Goddess/Half Squat

utkata konasana

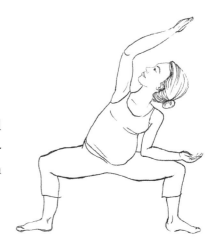

Benefits

Stretches through the hips, groins and chest while being stabilising and balancing. Strengthens through the thigh muscles.

How to

From standing with the front of the body parallel to the long edge of the mat, take a wide step, keeping both feet on the mat. Open the feet to an angle, as closely to parallel to the edge of the mat as possible. With hands on hips, soften into the knees. Knees need to stay tracking over the ankles. Thighs are as close to parallel to the ground as is comfortable. When ready, move hands into prayer position at the chest and on each exhale be aware of a deepening into the squat position. To modify, place hands onto the back of a chair or the wall for balance and support.

Options

Upper body side stretch (as pictured). Rest the flexed left arm onto the left leg and raise the right arm up towards the ceiling. Gaze up to the raised arm if balanced. Bring the upper body back to neutral on an inhalation and repeat on the opposite side.

Circle the arms with the breath. To build awareness of breath, keep legs static and from prayer position, on the inhalation raise arms up above the head and open the arms out in a wide circular movement, coming back through centre on the exhalation into prayer position.

Traditional. Lift your arms up, bending your elbows so they are at 90 degree angles, and open your palms away from you.

Calf stretch and strengthen. Lift the right heel on the inhalation and release on the exhalation. Repeat with the left heel on the next breath and alternate lifting the heels, breath by breath, while keeping the hands in prayer position at the front of the chest.

Standing

In Spanish, the word for labour is 'trabajar', which literally translated means *work*. In English, it is also another term for work... and work it often is.

Regardless of how each person experiences labour and the pain, preparing for labour and building a coping mindset can help someone to shift from suffering to acceptance. Incorporating asana from the standing series through each practice works well in preparation for birth.

By practising the asanas in the standing series, women are strengthening and preparing the body, while also energising themselves and releasing deep tension.

Modified Mountain Pose into Standing Side Stretch

Benefits

This asana stretches and releases through the side body and the intercostal muscles. This area can become compressed and tight during pregnancy, as the internal organs shift around and make space for the growing fetus and placenta.

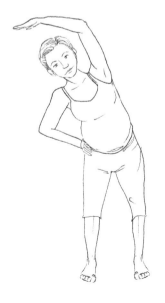

How to

From standing, place feet hip-width distance apart, with the feet either parallel or with heels slightly wider than the toes. Feet can be wider than hip-width distance if pressure is felt through the pelvis. Soften through the toes and be aware of the four corners of the soles of both feet evenly pressing down. Start with arms by the side and tuck through the pelvis.

On an inhalation, place the left hand onto the hip and extend the right arm towards the ceiling. On the exhalation, reach the fingertips of the right arm towards the left wall and keep the hips in line, facing forwards. Extend through the right side of the neck while keeping it long. Keep the biceps hugging the ears and the elbows as straight as possible. Hold for 5-10 breaths and return to standing by raising the stretched arm back through centre. Repeat with the left arm.

Options

Interlace both hands above the head and press the palms of the interlaced hands towards the ceiling. Keep the hands interlaced to stretch from side to side. Either move from side to side with each breath in and out, or hold the stretch on one side for five breaths and then the other side for five breaths.

Warrior 2

virabhadrasana 2

Benefits

In this asana, there are three elements that are built up and prepare women to be birth warriors. A warrior is ready for anything, without plan or attachment to outcome. The samurai warrior would practise and be ready at all times.

As birthing women, build up

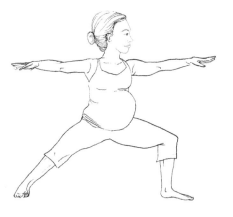

that sense of readiness through strength, focus and balance. The gaze is focused, you have strength through the legs and balance through the arms.

How to

From standing position, on an exhalation step the left foot towards the back of the mat at a 90 degree angle. (Make sure it is no wider than 90 degrees). If pelvic pain is present, shorten the stance and extend the front leg to a degree that is comfortable. Flex the left knee in line with the right heel without dropping the knee inwards.

On an inhalation, raise arms up so they are parallel to the mat, with palms facing down. Keep the focus and gaze through the middle fingers of the left hand. Hold for 5 breaths. To release, extend the left knee on an inhalation, releasing arms to the side of the body on the exhalation. Repeat on the opposite side.

Options

Dynamic. Create movement through the arms and shoulders by keeping the legs steady. On each inhalation bring the hands together in front of the chest into prayer position, and on the exhalation return arms to the parallel position. Repeat five times.

Modified Side Stretch
modified parsvottanasana

Benefits

A nurturing, heart-opening posture. Improves balance while stretching through the hamstrings in the back of the legs. Also works as a chest opener to create space and openness through the front of the body, which may be compromised during pregnancy with the increased weight of the breasts and abdomen.

How to

From standing position, step the right foot back about a metre/3 feet, with the left foot pointing forward and right foot at a 45 degree angle. Straighten through both legs or keep the front knee bent if there is too much strain through the back of the leg. Take arms behind the back into reverse namaskar, touching opposite elbows with the arms bent, or else in- 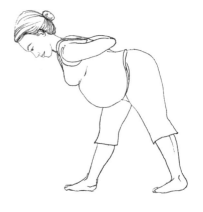 terlace hands behind the back with straight arms. Some students may prefer to remain upright.

If moving forward, on the inhalation open through the chest and on the exhalation fold forward, taking care not to compress through the abdomen by folding further forward than the height of the hips. Hold for 5 breaths, and on an inhalation return to standing. Release the hands on the exhalation. Repeat on the opposite side.

Experienced practitioners can move into standing split (Urdhva Prasarita Ekapadasana).

NOTE: Full parsvottasana compresses through the abdomen and is contraindicated through pregnancy.

Side Angle
utthita parsvokasana

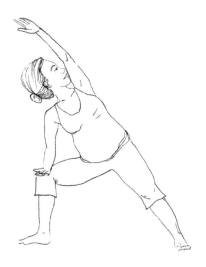

Benefits

Strengthens and stretches the legs, knees, and ankles. Stretches the groins, spine, waist, chest and lungs, and shoulders.

How to

Start with the left leg forward in Warrior 2 stance, with the front knee flexed. Rest the flexed left forearm onto the left thigh. Raise the right arm up towards the ceiling and stretch the fingertips over the head. Ensure the abdomen is not compressed with any forward folding. Hold for five breaths. To release, use the left hand resting on the knee as support to return to centre. Repeat on the other side.

Standing Chest Openers

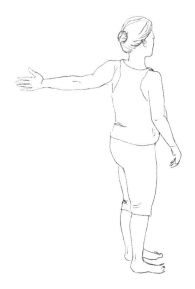

Benefits

Releases through the shoulders. Releases through the pectoral muscles and through the front of the body and neck. Great for pregnancy so as to release any forward shoulder rolling from the increased weight. Beneficial post birth too, after feeding and holding the baby forward.

How to

Start by facing into the wall with feet hip-width distance apart, with the right shoulder next to the wall. Raise the extended right arm and press the palm into the wall at shoulder height.

Take the left hand behind the back, with palm facing out, and pivot both feet 90 degrees so the right hand stays on the wall and the body rotates to face the opposite direction. Every exhalation, open the shoulder a little more and take gaze away from the body. Keep the gaze forward if there are any neck issues.

Hold for at least 10 breaths. To release, rotate the body back to face the wall, release the arm and then repeat on the opposite side. After both sides, either do shoulder shrugs or circle through the shoulders to release.

Modified Down Dog

Benefits

Stretches through the hamstrings and releases through the mid and upper back. A supported asana that can be practised throughout pregnancy, and is also a position that is fantastic for labour.

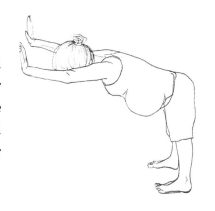

How to

Place both hands on wall at shoulder-width distance and step feet back to hip-width distance. Ensure hands are at hip height or higher (as illustrated). Release through the head and the neck and press into the heels while drawing the tail bone back. Hold for 20 breaths. To release, draw the body upright and step towards the wall, creating a cushion for the head with the forearms. I like to repeat this position in a class.

Modify by leaning onto the back of a chair, ensuring the shoulders are not lower than the hips. Placing hands wider than shoulder-width gives greater release through the upper back.

Standing Calf Stretch

Benefits
Releases through the calf muscles and helps to maintain body mobility. Practise at home if suffering from leg cramps.

How to
Stand facing the wall and press both hands into the wall, with the elbows flexed. Step the right foot back and press into the heel while bending into the left knee. Hold for 5-10 breaths and release. Repeat with the left leg. If the calves are particularly tight, gently pump heel up and down of the extended leg to release before the static hold.

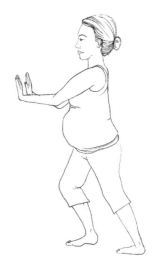

Options
The calf stretch can be practised from a hands and knees position (see p.64).

Pelvic Tilt

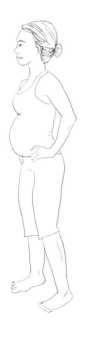

Benefits

Builds awareness of the pelvic floor muscles and how to engage and release them. Releasing the pelvic floor is necessary through birth. This asana connects movement with breath.

How to

Standing at the front of the mat, place feet hip-width distance apart and parallel. With hands on the hips, bend into the knees and on an exhalation, engage the pelvic floor and draw the front of the pelvis upwards. On the inhalation, soften and release to neutral. Be aware when releasing that the pelvic floor is not being pushed downwards. Repeat 10 times. This can also be practised against the wall for support by placing palms on the wall at shoulder height.

Options

This can be done in a supine position (see p. 103).

Hip Circling

From the pelvic tilt position, keep the soles of the feet pressing into the mat while circling the hips in one direction for 10 breaths. Then circle for 10 breaths in the other direction.

This movement softens through the pelvis and builds awareness of movement with breath.

Arms/Shoulders

The arms and shoulders asanas offer wonderful sequencing opportunities and can be used for warm up, woven through a class or practised towards the end of the class to build up mental stamina.

The asanas from the arm/shoulders series asana can be practised in a seated, kneeling or standing position.

Eagle Arms

garudasana

Benefits

Releases through the wrists and shoulders and opens through the shoulder blades. Ensure wrists are neutral if suffering carpal tunnel.

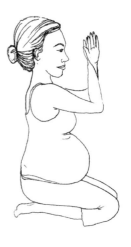

How to

Extend arms and cross arms at the elbow. Bend your elbows, and then raise your forearms perpendicular to the floor. Wrap your arms and hands, and press your palms together (or as close as possible). If you are unable to get the palms to touch, have the backs of the hands touching. If standing, have both feet on the mat, hip-width distance apart.

N.B. The regular garudasana legs are contraindicated, as there can be too much abdominal compression from the position and from trying to hold balance.

Arms Outstretched and Circling

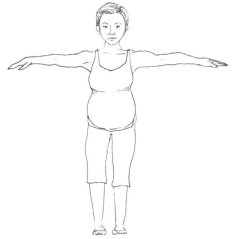

Benefits

Stretches and tones through the arms and can be done my most people. Gives rotation through the shoulder cuffs. Builds strength and endurance through the body and mind connection. Increases circulation to the wrists and fingers.

How to

Extend arms with hands in line with the shoulders, and have palms facing down. Begin with a small circular motion through the arms. Follow your breath and in a rhythm, feel the circles slowly getting bigger. Build up the intensity by widening the size of the circles. Change direction to decrease the size of the circle, coming back to the small circles you began with. Release arms down to the side of the body.

Options

Circling of arms above head. Raise arms to full extension, with palms facing upwards. On an inhalation, palms meet above the head at the end of the 'in' breath. On the exhalation, circle arms around and down, and at the end of the exhalation meet hands in prayer through the heart centre. Repeat as many times as you like, to build awareness of movement with breath.

Arms clasped behind back. Interlace fingers behind the back and draw shoulder blades in towards each other on the exhalation. Lift clasped hands towards the ceiling without dropping body forward or hunching through the shoulders.

Extension and flexion. Turn palms towards the ceiling. On an inhalation, bend elbows and tap fingertips onto the top of the shoulder. On exhalation, draw the elbows up towards the ceiling without drawing the shoulders up to the ears. On the inhalation release elbows and on the exhalation extend arms fully. This is one cycle. Repeat as many times as you like.

Hitchhiking Arms

Benefits

Rotation through the shoulder joints.

I learned the hitchhiking arms asana from a kundalini teacher in Santa Barbara, California.

A great asana both to build up endurance and to explore the mind for an "I don't want to do this anymore" mindset, so have students push through that. The sensations through the shoulders can become quite strong; this is a 'stay in' asana. Find the strength within to stay in it and not give up.

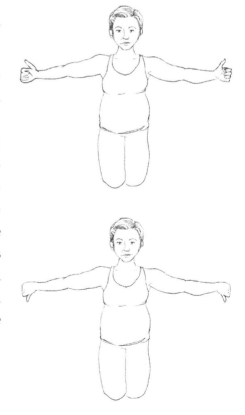

It makes ideal preparation for the mental endurance needed for labour and birth.

How to

From a sitting or kneeling position, extend arms out to the side. Create a fist and have the thumbs sticking up, as if hitchhiking.

Rotate through the shoulders, and on the inhalation point the thumbs up. On the exhalation point the thumbs down.

Continue the movement for at least a minute.

Balancing

The balance series includes asanas that are opportunities to practise staying in the centre and letting go of control. Physically, the centre of gravity shifts during pregnancy and so it is not uncommon for women to feel out of balance during this time.

Mentally and emotionally, there are many shifts in pregnancy that can also affect physical balance. Experiencing the physical being out of balance can give greater insight into the deeper layers within.

Sometimes people hold their breath as a way of trying to keep their balance. Keep awareness on a steady flow of breath as the body maintains balance.

Work with drishti by finding a still point to focus the gaze on before entering an asana. This can help keep the body become more centred and balanced. Try closing the eyes for a second or two in a balancing asana to explore the effectiveness of keeping the gaze still and steady. If needed, the balance series can be practised leaning the hands or fingertips against a wall.

Quads Stretch and Preparation for Dancer's Pose

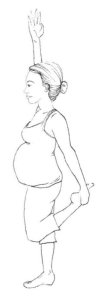

Benefits

Releases tension and stiffness through the front of the legs and increases flexibility and circulation.

Starting in this position before moving into Dancers Pose gives women the opportunity to explore their balance, since this shifts and changes through pregnancy.

How to

Start in the neutral standing position and on an inhalation, flex the right knee and take hold of the foot from the outside edge. Draw the heel in towards the buttocks while keeping the knees in line. Raise the left arm up towards the ceiling in preparation for dancers pose as illustrated, and rest on the hip or touch the fingertips on the wall for extra balance support.

Continue to Dancer's Pose after holding for 5 breaths, or release and repeat on the opposite side.

Dancer's Pose

natarajasana

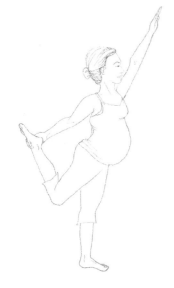

Benefits

Improves balance while stretching through the legs, chest and shoulders and strengthening through the ankles and legs. I find this such a graceful asana; although some women through pregnancy feel they have lost some of their gracefulness, by practising this asana, they can connect and embody that grace of a dancer.

How to

From the quads stretch position, on an exhalation bend forward through the hips as you press the foot into the hand, extending the lifted leg. Either have the hand raised as illustrated or touch the fingertips on a wall to support the outstretched hand for balance.

Ensure there is no compression through the abdomen, and with the balance and forward movement be careful to allow the breath full movement. Hold for 5 breaths and release by drawing the body back to centre on an inhalation. Repeat on the opposite side.

Half Moon Pose
ardha chandrasana

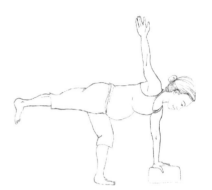

Benefits

This is an advanced posture for pregnancy and generally for the more experienced yoga students.

Builds balance and strength through
the legs.

Opens through the chest and shoulders while building stamina and endurance.

How to

From standing, step one foot back approximately 1 metre (4 feet), raise arms up parallel to the mat, and bend into the front knee. On an exhalation, release the front hand down towards the block or mat as you raise the leg on the same side up. Flex through the foot of the lifted leg. Release by dropping the leg down and bring the arm back to the side.

Make sure to practise both sides of the body. Start by focusing the gaze downwards and only shift their gaze if stable.

Using a block can reduce compression through the abdomen and offer more support to balance. Using the back of a chair instead of a block can give extra support.

Tree Pose
vriksasana

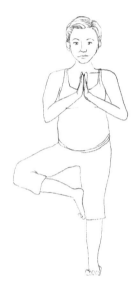

Benefits

Builds balance, focus and clarity. Opens through the hips.

How to

From standing position, with hands on the hips or touching on a wall for balance, shift weight into left foot while externally rotating the flexed right knee. If unable to lift the foot off the ground, touch the toes on the floor for balance. With the added relaxin the ligaments through the knees can become looser, so take care that the foot is placed either above or below the knee, and not pushing directly into the side of the knee.

Arms can stay on the hips or press together at heart centre as illustrated. Express arms in other ways if desired, towards the sky to receive energy or point fingers towards the earth to ground. Take arms behind the back in reverse prayer, for heart opening and emotional release.

Seated

Patanjali's yoga sutras tell us that asana should be steady and comfortable (2.46 Stkira Sukham Asanam)[27]. The seated series are a preparation to find comfort and stability through the body. Working on this series during pregnancy builds this awareness of stability through the body, mind and emotions.

In the early stages of pregnancy, it can be beneficial to sit in easy seat pose with the eyes closed and practise breath awareness. I have found that towards the later stages of pregnancy, many women prefer to end their class in a seated meditative position.

When I went on my first Vipassana 10-day course at 32 weeks' pregnant with my first son, I found that my belly's shape and size gave my back great support, while the relaxin worked through my hips, creating a very comfortable seat to be able to cope with the discomfort that was present at times over the course of those 10 days as I sat and meditated.

Easy Seat
sukhasana

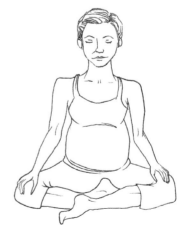

Benefits

A centered and stable position to enter into meditation or pranayama. Sitting in this position strengthens through the back and stretches through the knees.

How to

From a seated position on the floor, cross the legs and draw knees towards the mat. If hips are lower than the knees, sit on a folded blanket or cushion to elevate the hips.

In easy posture you can have the hands on knees and palms facing up or down. Palms facing up signifies giving and receiving, while the palms down signifies abiding and calm.

Warm up options from easy seat

If unable to sit cross-legged, the warm up movements can be practised standing, kneeling, with legs out straight, in gomukasana legs or sitting on a chair. It is important to ensure the spine is not slumped for these movements.

Shoulders

Interlace the hands, straighten arms and raise them above the head. Have the palms facing towards the ceiling. On an exhale, draw the interlaced hands forward and press into the palms. Gently curve the spine here.

Chest

Interlace the hands behind the back and extend the arms. Take care to keep the spine upright to stretch through the pectoral muscles.

Side body

On the inhalation, raise and extend the right arm. With the palm facing the head, on the exhalation, reach the fingertips across, keeping the shoulders away from the ears. Soften through the head and draw the left ear towards the left shoulder. Place the left hand on the mat, with fingers pointing away from the body. Bend into the elbow of the left hand to deepen if flexibility allows. Hold for 5-10 breaths. To release, on an inhalation raise the right arm and on the exhalation release the right arm down beside the body. Repeat with the left arm.

Ankle joints

Extend the legs in front at hip-width distance. Rotate the feet in a circular motion in a clockwise direction and then the opposite way. Paddle the feet in flexion and extension.

Modified Seated Forward Stretch

Benefits

Stretches through the torso and hips and builds awareness of body changes and potential limitations through pregnancy.

How to

From the easy seated pose, on inhalation raise both arms above the head. On exhalation extend the arms in front and touch the fingertips or palms on the mat. Walk the fingertips slowly to the right and then back through centre and towards the left to gain some gentle upper body movement. Take care to avoid compression through the abdomen.

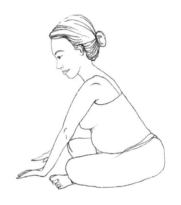

Neck Stretches

Benefits

Releases tension through the neck and upper torso. Increases neck mobility and can reduce headaches and tension through the face and jaw.

For all movements through the neck, avoid any jerky movements of the head. Be sensitive and only go as deeply into the stretch as is comfortable.

How to

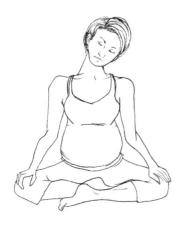

From seated position, start on the left side. On an exhalation soften the left ear down towards the left shoulder while keeping the shoulders in line. To deepen the stretch, on exhalation release the left shoulder downwards slightly and be aware of the release through the neck. Hold for 5-10 breaths. Release on an inhalation by raising the head back to centre. Repeat on the right side.

Forwards and backwards

On an exhalation, draw the chin gently down towards the chest. Hold for 5-10 breaths as the back of the neck lengthens. To release, on an inhalation bring the head to centre and hold for a breath. On an exhalation release the head backwards and hold for 5-10 breaths. Soften through the jaw while in this position by moving the jaw from side to side. Release on an inhalation by bringing the head back to centre.

Left and right rotation

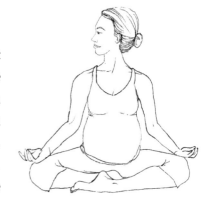

From centre, start by looking out towards the left shoulder. Keep the head upright and rotate the chin towards the left shoulder. With each exhale move the chin a little further, taking care to not crunch into the neck. Hold for 5-10 breaths, and release the head back to centre on an inhalation. Repeat on the right side.

Wide-Legged Forward Fold

upavista konasana

Benefits

Stretches through the adductors—the muscles through the inner thigh—and through the hamstrings at the back of the thighs.

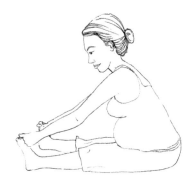

If suffering from pain in the pubic symphysis do not take the legs out wider than hip-width distance. Rest hands on shins to avoid compression through the forward fold.

How to

From a seated position with legs straight out in front, take hands behind the back to start, palms facing down, with fingers pointing towards the body. Open the legs as wide as possible and start to draw the torso forward slightly. If there is a stretch through the inside of the legs while the hands are behind the back, stay here. If there is a need to go deeper, take the hands forward and walk the fingertips forward.

Make sure the fold is from the hips and not the waist, and keep the spine tall. To support knees, place a block beneath each knee. To raise hips, sit on a folded blanket or cushion to reduce pressure on knees.

Take care not to compress through the abdomen. This may reduce how far forward the more flexible people may go. Hold for 10-20 breaths.

The aim here is not to go as deep as possible but to explore the body and how it opens with each breath. Holding this pose for a couple of minutes gives women the chance to work with their breath and movement. Advise them to notice the space their inhale creates, and move into the space on their exhale.

Modified Head to Knee Pose
janu sirsasana

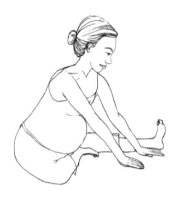

Benefits

Stretches through the spine, shoulders, hamstrings and groin.

The aim here is to lengthen hamstrings (not get the head to the knee).

How to

From a wide-legged seated position, flex through the right knee and place the right foot on the inside of the left thigh. For people who can't do this, place the right foot onto the shin of the left leg. Place hands forward as illustrated or take hands over to the extended left, either onto the shin or hold onto the foot. Ensure the abdomen is not compressed. To release, on an inhale lift through the torso. Extend both legs and repeat on the opposite side.

Option

Back bend. Increase energy and add a back bend here by placing the sole of the left leg's foot on the mat. Place the right hand behind the back, with palm facing down and fingers pointing away from the body. Lift the hips off the mat on an inhalation and hold for 5 breaths. Release on an exhale.

Seated Open Side Stretch

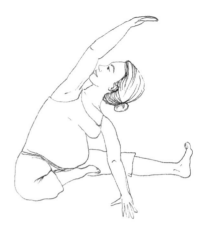

Benefits

Releases and stretches through the ribs and intercostal muscles.

How to

From a seated position, extend the left leg and flex the foot. Bend through the right knee and take the right foot to the inside of the left thigh.

Stretch through the upper arm and side body while keeping the left hand forward to create space, and opening through the chest. The supporting left hand can also rest on the shin or foot of the extended leg, if flexibility allows. Hold for 5-10 breaths.

Release on an inhalation by raising through the torso. Repeat on the opposite side. If there is compression through the abdomen on the side stretch, point fingertips of the raised arm towards the ceiling.

Option (add this before changing sides):

Deep thigh stretch

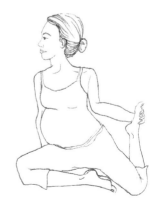

From the seated open side stretch position, with the upper body in neutral, take the left hand behind the body and bend through the extended leg. Take hold of the foot of that leg and draw the heel in towards the buttocks. Keep the chest open and avoid any rounding through the shoulders. Release on exhalation and repeat on the opposite side.

Cow Face Pose

gomukasana

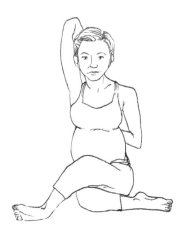

Benefits

Opens and releases through the muscles across the chest. Stretches ankles, hips and thighs, shoulders, armpits, and triceps, and extends through latissimus dorsi.

This seated position can be a good option for students with pubic symphysis. The opening through the chest and front body is also ideal through pregnancy. Practise the arm movements daily, at least once on each side, if spending a lot of time in front of a computer.

How to

From a seated position extend both legs. Flex the left leg and place the foot near the right buttock. Flex the right leg over the left leg, with the knees on top of each other as closely as possible. Ensure the hip bones are even. On an inhalation raise the right arm and on the exhalation take the hand down the spine. Use the left hand to press into the elbow and, without curving through the spine, take the left hand behind the back, taking hold of the right hand. Stay here for 5-10 breaths and then release arms and legs. Repeat on the opposite side.

The arms can stay resting on top of the knee if the person has high blood pressure or are not comfortable lifting arms above the head.

Back Bends

Back bends can be relieving through pregnancy, although they do need to be practised with caution. Deep back bending can de-stabilise the sacroiliac joint and/or overstretch through the abdomen. Many of the traditional backbends are contraindicated through pregnancy.

Continuing with the modified back bend positions through pregnancy can be helpful in relieving tension through the spine. It also encourages opening through the chest and the front of the body, including the heart centre.

Modified Camel

ustrasana

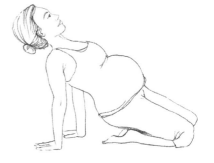

Benefits

An energising back bend which also opens up through the front of the body and chest. Releases through the neck. Stretches through the quadriceps.

I often see regular practitioners continuing with full camel all through their pregnancy. They have the flexibility, however be aware that doing this can overstretch the abdominals and can cause separation problems during pregnancy or post birth. Additionally, the sacroiliac joints can become overly compressed.

How to

From a kneeling position, take both hands to the lower back, with fingers pointing towards the ground and draw the elbows towards each other. Can be practised kneeling in toe tuck or with the tops of their feet flat on the mat. To deepen, place hands onto the mat with fingers pointing away from the body as illustrated, or pointing towards the body if preferred. Hold for 5-10 breaths. To release, one at a time place hands back to the lower back and draw forward. Move into a wide-legged child's pose for at least 5 breaths.

Options

Alternate left and right sides. Instead of taking both hands back, from the kneeling position, start by placing the left hand with the palm down behind and have fingers pointing away from the body. Raise up the right arm and look up towards the right fingertips. On an exhalation release the body back to centre and on the inhalation repeat on the other side. To deepen, when the hand is pressing behind, lift up through the hips. Either have a static back bend by holding for between 5-10 breaths on each side or alternate sides breath-to-breath.

This can be a static or dynamic asana. There is also the choice of how deep to go in this position.

Bridge Pose
setu bandha sarvangasana

Benefits

Stretches through the hips, chest, spine and legs. Strengthens through the back, and can build awareness of how to stabilise with engagement through the pelvic floor.

Recommended for trimesters one and two only. For the third trimester substitute with an alternate back bend or standing pelvic tilts (p. 84)

A supported bridge can be practised for people with breech babies but this is not something I teach in class. I direct people to do further investigation and there are many resources available with this information. Spinning Babies (**www.spinningbabies.com**) is a great resource for optimal fetal positioning.

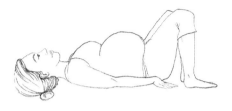

Preparation for bridge pose

How to

From a supine position, flex the knees, with feet flat on the mat at hip-width distance apart. With feet pressing evenly into the mat, inhale to lift the hips up. Place hands next to the body with palms facing down. Hold for 5-10 breaths. Release the hips to the mat on exhalation.

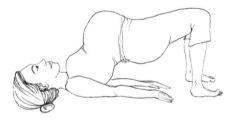

Full bridge pose

Options

Supine pelvic tilts. Make this a dynamic movement through the hips, moving with the breath. Inhale to lift and exhale to release.

Transverse abdominal strengthening. From the supine starting position, with knees bent lift alternate heels, with toes pressing into the mat. Repeat 10 times on each side.

Side lying

The side lying series is not a traditional set of yoga asana and are closer to pilates movements than the traditional hatha poses. Including them in pregnancy yoga diversifies the options for women to increase strength, engagement and movement through the gluteal muscles and the legs, while being supported by the floor so as to avoid unnecessary strain through the back. Properly engaging the gluteal muscles also supports the health of the pelvic floor muscles, as there is activation through these stabilising muscles. These are subtle repetitive movements to maximise the building of strength, without strain.

Straight Leg Raises

Benefits

Helps to strengthen the gluteal muscles which are important stabilisers, particularly in pregnancy when a lot of core strength is compromised.

Can be a good preparation for the side-lying birth position.

How to

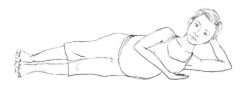

Starting on the left side of the body, extend legs and support the torso with the upper arm. Head can be propped up and supported by the lower arm, or have the arm extended and flat on the mat, with head resting on the upper arm.

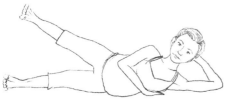

Upper arm can be resting on the mat for support or resting on the top hip for a stronger posture.

On an inhalation lift the right leg while keeping the hips in line. Avoid any roll forward through the right hip. On an exhalation release the leg back to starting position. Repeat 10 times. On release, give a little self massage through the glutes if needed.

Roll over to repeat on the opposite side in any way that is comfortable.

N.B. If adding any of the below options, do all the variations on the left side of the body before moving to lie on the right side of the body.

Clam Leg Raises with bent legs (and variations)

Benefits

Strengthens the gluteus maximus and medius, which adds to core support and back strength.

At the end of the reps, give a little self massage to release the gluteal region. If suffering from pubic symphysis pain, only perform the option with knees pressed together.

How to

From the side lying position, bend both knees to a 90 degree angle. Rest head on the outstretched lower arm and rest the hand on upper hip or abdomen. Repeat as many variations on one side as desired before changing sides and then follow the same sequence on the other side.

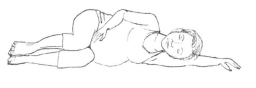

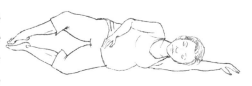

Options

Feet together, open knees. On an exhalation keep the inside edges of the feet contacted and lift the upper knee. Making sure to keep the hips stable. Release to neutral on the inhalation. Repeat 10 times. Roll over and repeat on the opposite side.

Knees together, raise feet. Keeping the knees pressing in together, lift through the upper foot on an exhalation. Taking care to not rock back through the hips.

Lift both foot and knee. Keep the foot and knee of the upper leg in line and on the exhalation lift the bent leg (imagine there is a cup on the shin to keep it straight). Release to neutral on the inhalation. Repeat 10 times. Roll over and repeat on the opposite side.

Hips

The hip joints are ball and socket joints located at the juncture of the leg and pelvis. The hip joints are the second largest weight-bearing joints in the body, after the knee. With the additional weight through pregnancy and the impact through the joints from relaxin, these joints can be put under extra pressure and strain. Maintaining and releasing these joints is helpful during pregnancy and in preparation for birth.

It is ideal to practise the hip opening series after the body has warmed up, when there is time to soften and sink into the joints.

Seated Hip Opener

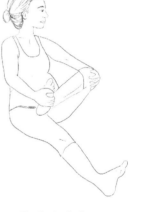

Benefits

Opens hips while increasing flexibility. Also encourages alignment through the pelvis, which can become distorted during pregnancy.

How to

From seated, lift the top leg, keep it bent and have one hand supporting the knee and the other hand, the foot.

Rock the baby

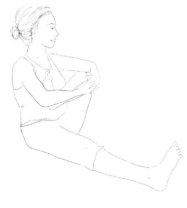

Draw the shin in towards the chest, and if there is the flexibility, clasp the hands so the knee and foot are supported by the elbows. With a rocking motion, move the leg from side to side, releasing through the hips. Repeat on the other side.

At any stage, if not possible to clasp the hands, keep supporting the foot and knee

Cradle the baby

with the hands to make the rocking motion.

Butterfly
baddha konasana

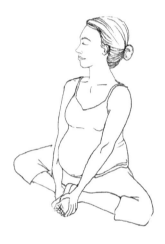

Benefits

This asana can assist opening through the hips and can help soften the attachments through the pelvic bones. Through pregnancy try to sit in this pose for at least 5 minutes a day. Incorporate this position into daily life. If watching TV, sit on the floor in this pose as a way to avoid the couch slump posture. This slumping has been shown to affect a baby's position.

The Belly Mapping workbook by Gail Tully and her website 'spinningbabies.com' are both resources that have a range of information available on optimal fetal positioning.

How to

Start with legs straight out in front and bring the soles of the feet in to touch. While bending through the knees, bring the heels in towards the body. Hold onto the feet with the hands as shown. Place hands on the shins with palms facing down if it is not possible to fully bend forward to hold the feet. The feet further from the body is more gentle, while closer to the pelvis is a stronger position.

If the hips feel very tight in this position, sit on a cushion or folded blanket to raise the pelvis. Can also be practised in a supine position with a bolster propping up the torso.

Pigeon Pose

kapotasana

Benefits

Gives a deep stretch through the glutes and the psoas (long lumbar muscle). Can help relieve sciatic pain.

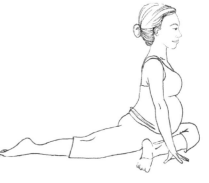

I don't teach this asana in every class. It depends on who is in the class and how experienced they are with yoga. I find for the women in third trimester and/or are quite new to yoga that this asana can be too strong and overly uncomfortable. As with all the asana, also have women check in with themselves and work to their capacity.

How to

From hands and knees position, bring the right knee forward towards the right wrist. Place the ankle at a point in front of the left hip. The more parallel the right shin is to the top of the mat, the stronger the posture. Stay upright and use the hands as pictured to support to avoid compressing through the abdomen. If folding forward, use bolsters across the chest for support to avoid compression through the abdomen. Ensure the right hip on the mat. If the right hip lifts, bend the left leg as much as needed to have the hip rest on the mat.

To modify, sit on a chair and cross the right leg over the left leg, with the right ankle resting on the left knee. Press the right knee towards the mat for a release through the piriformis and/or sciatic pain.

Happy Baby Pose
ananda balasana

Benefits

Can relieve lower back pain by releasing through the lower back and sacrum, while opening the hips, inner thighs and groin.

In any practice, this asana is always optional, as some women become nauseous lying on their back, even for a very short time. Not recommended in third trimester.

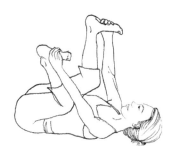

How to

From a supine position, open the knees slightly wider than the torso and bring them up toward the armpits. Hold onto the outside or inside edges of the feet or the shins for 3-5 breaths. Rock from side to side and do not stay static for more than 10 seconds.

Relaxation

savasana

Savasana traditionally is a time when
the practice you've done integrates
through the body, and this is also true
in prenatal yoga.

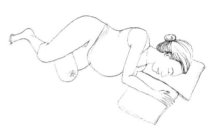

Finding deep relaxation through
pregnancy creates a clearer environment for the fetus to develop through
their own koshas. Emotions travel as hormones through the bloodstream and this blood flow crosses over through the placenta to the
fetus. The fetus will experience all of the emotions that are experienced
by the mother.

Practising deep rest is an important element of birth preparation. In
labour it is the time between the contractions that is as important as the
contractions themselves. It's a time to re-centre and balance in preparation for the next moment of the birth.

The relaxation asanas can be done on their own or towards the end
of the practice.

Legs Up Wall Pose
viparita karani

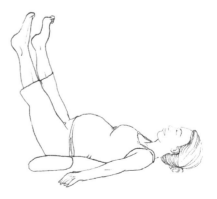

Benefits

Can relieve lower back pain and
release tension through the legs.
Calms through the nervous system
and is an inversion. This can be

powerful through pregnancy, when women carry a lot of stress about unknowns. The asana gives space for a shift in perspective.

If women are getting swollen ankles/edema from fluid retention, then this can relieve swelling.

How to

Place a folded blanket, cushion or bolster at the wall and from a seated position facing the wall, move into a supine position with feet on the wall. Press into the feet to lift the hips onto the prop. The prop can sit across the hips or sacrum. Extend legs up the wall.

If extending the legs creates discomfort, keep knees bent with feet pressing into the wall. Hands rest beside the body or on abdomen to connect to baby. Hold for a few minutes. To release, bend through the knees and when ready roll over to one side.

Stay on side for 5-10 breaths (or longer if moving straight to savasana) before moving to an upright position.

Supported Reclining Butterfly
supta baddha konasana

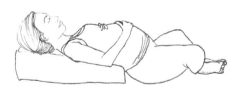

Benefits

A deeply relaxing position that releases and stretches through the pelvis and hips.

Place an eye mask over the eyes to reduce the sensory input.

Can be practised at the beginning of class or at the end, or both!

How to

Place a bolster (can also use a block under the bolster for greater height) vertically on the mat and lie over the bolster. Bring soles of the feet together and draw the heels in towards the body. Feet closer to the body is stronger, taking the heels further away is gentler. If there is pain through the knees, place props under the knees for added support.

Side Lying Pose
savasana

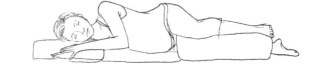

Benefits

Deeply restorative and relaxing.

Practise savasana for at least five minutes in a comfortable position at the end of the practice. Side lying takes the pressure off the vena cava (the vein that runs slightly to the right of the spine, responsible for returning blood from the legs back to the heart), which can compress in the full supine position.

Traditionally, women have been advised to lie on the left side of the body, however, the current recommendation is to choose the more comfortable side at the time.

Avoid the prop opening through the legs if suffering from pubic symphysis disorder.

How to

Lie down on the preferred side of the body and place a prop under the head or the bottom arm to support the neck and spine. Place a bolster or cushion between the knees to support the top leg. At the end of the five minutes, or longer if desired, gently move through the fingers and toes to awaken the body. Have a stretch through the arms and legs and come up to a seated position to close the practice.

Chapter NINE

Partner Asanas

Partner Asanas

Partner asanas are a wonderful way for people to connect and prepare for birth. Take dedicated partner classes or include one or two partner asana in a prenatal class. Introduce the asana and instructions carefully, as people have varying flexibility, conditions and experience. Ensure that the person assisting works within their partner's limits.

These are great practice for people to support and feel supported... to touch and connect. These postures build trust, as both practitioners need to trust the other to be able to fully release in the positions. The partner series gives an opportunity to build breath awareness and also connection and support ideas as they move into different positions together.

Although only the pregnant woman is giving birth, have their partners experience all the asana. It is good for the women to experience the support role and for their partners to experience the positions their partners may labour and birth in.

Supported Partner Squat

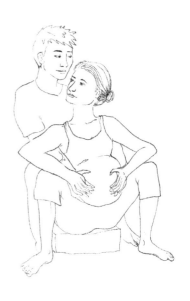

Benefits

This is a supportive and opening position; it encourages deep connection and provides a space to hold and be held.

I have heard that for birth this position can place a lot of pressure on the perineum and may tear more, but through labour this position encourages opening through the pelvis and is supportive and nurturing.

This position can work well in a birthing pool through labour, where partners can either be in the pool or out of it, supporting from behind.

I would not include this position in a general prenatal class, just in specific birth partner classes or sessions.

How to

Partners sit on a chair or stool up against a wall and place a bolster or folded blanket in front of them. The person squatting will sit on the prop, facing away from their partner as illustrated, and open through their knees. Supporting partners can place their hands around baby / belly. There is the opportunity here for eye contact, which supports oxytocin production, and for deep nurturing touch.

Partner Warrior 2

Benefits

Builds strength, stamina and endurance, with the added element of support and connection.

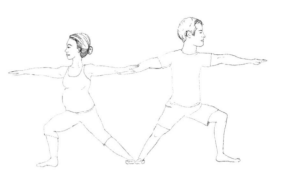

Works well in a general prenatal class or a specific partner class.

How to

Stand facing the same direction as your partner and take a wide step, keeping the outside edge of the feet closest to each other touching. Hold onto the forearms of each other's arms on the same side as feet that are touching. Turn the foot that is not touching out to a 90 degree angle and flex the knee so it does not extend past the ankle. Raise and extend the free arm parallel to the mat, with the palm facing down. Hold for 5-10 breaths. Release by extending through the bent knee and releasing the arms. Then swap sides and repeat.

Partner Child's Pose with Massage

Benefits

Nurturing and relaxing position. The added massage can be releasing and supportive.

In labour this position is often used in between contractions. The touch and release from the partner can encourage oxytocin production.

How to

From hands and knees position, widen knees to either side of the mat and draw the big toes towards each other to touch if possible. On an exhalation, draw hips back towards the heels and slide hands out towards the front of the mat. Lengthen through the arms on the inhalation and further release hips on the exhalation. Keep hips high

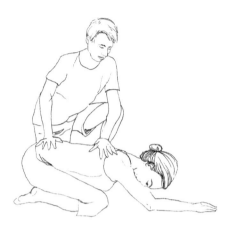

in the air if there is any pressure through the abdomen, which is more common during the later stages of pregnancy.

If it is not comfortable extending the arms out in front, create a cushion with the hands on top of each other for the forehead to rest on.

Partner to find a comfortable position and place both hands on the lower back or the tailbone, and press down. Working with their partner's breath and starting off with gentle pressure, increasing as they work with their partner to find the right amount of pressure.

Partner Supported Modified Down Dog with Massage

Benefits

A favoured labouring position, this is great practice for labour. In this position there is access to the lower back and sacrum. In labour, the use of a heat pack in this position can also be soothing. Can be practised at the wall or leaning on something to support.

Partners need to be aware of their own body mechanics and find ways to support without injuring themselves. If a lot of pressure is needed they can take the lunge position to build their strength rather

than just using their arms. Builds
communication about what works
and what doesn't, which is beneficial before birth.

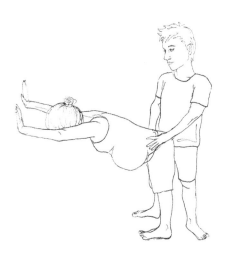

How to

Place both hands on wall, at
shoulder-width distance, and step
feet back to hip-width distance.
Ensure hands are at hip height
or higher (as illustrated). Release
through the head and the neck
and press into the heels while drawing the tail bone back. Partners can
gently massage through the lower back or shoulders, or else press into
the tail bone or the buttocks, working with their partner to check pressure and position while also taking care with their own body positioning. Hold for 20 breaths.

To release, draw the body upright and step towards the wall, creating a fusion for the head with the forearms. Swap partners. It can be
beneficial for the pregnant woman to experience the support role and
the potential demands that will be placed on her partner through their
support role during labour.

Modify by leaning onto the back of a chair, ensuring the shoulders
are not lower than the hips. Placing hands wider than shoulder width
gives greater release through the upper back.

Partner Tree

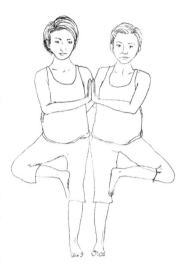

Benefits

Balancing and supportive position. This is a fun asana in a general class.

How to

Standing next to your partner, with arms around each others' waists, flex the knees of the outside legs and externally rotate. Find a point to focus the gaze on that does not move. Place the feet on the ankles, shins or above the knees on the thighs. Bring your outside arms to the middle, and touch palms in the prayer position. Hold for 5-10 breaths. Release, swap positions and repeat on the other side.

Partner Sway and Circling of Hips

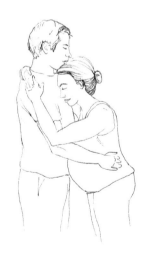

Benefits

This is a connected and nurturing position that I teach to birth couples. Not an asana I would include in a general asana class. Encourage this position at home; a soothing and gentle way to connect each day, especially when the due date is approaching. A wonderful position through labour. Partners can massage through the lower back in this position.

How to

Standing and facing each other, the pregnant woman reaches her arms around her partner's shoulders and he places his hands at her lower back. Finding own rhythm, rock gently from side to side or in gentle circular motion. Choose a song or two to sway and rock to.

Partner Seated and Standing Twist

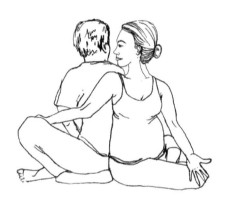

Benefits

Connected movement that opens and releases through the chest and upper back.

How to

Sit in easy seat, back to back, and both start with the right hand. On an inhalation, place the right hand with the palm facing down on the partners right thigh or knee (depending on reach). Open through the upper body while keeping the abdomen facing forward. Hold for 5-10 breaths, and release on an exhalation. Repeat with the left arm.

Partner Wide-legged Forward Fold

Benefits

Supports deeper release through the inner thighs. Builds awareness of movement with breath with partner.

How to

Sit on the mat across from each other, extend and widen the legs. Depending on leg length, either place the soles of the feet on each other or have the person with shorter legs place the soles of their feet on the inner ankles of

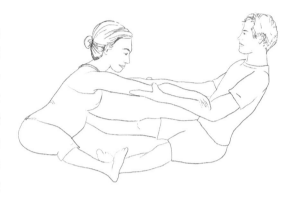

their partners. Both extend arms and take hold of each others wrists, forearms or elbows, depending on reach and flexibility. One partner softens backwards while the other draws forward. The person leaning backwards needs to listen to their partner's cues as to how far forward they can come, since they are the ones receiving the supported stretch.

Hold for 5-10 breaths, working with the breath of the partner folding forward, deepening with each of their exhalations. Draw up on an inhalation and take 3 full breaths together at centre before repeating with the opposite roles.

Chapter TEN

Pranayama

Pranayama

Building an awareness of the breath is integral to all yoga practices and plays an important part of the prenatal yoga practice. Through pregnancy and birth, breath can be a grounding anchor. Physiologically, it can activate the calm and connection system. Breath awareness also allows people to focus on one point and keep centred.

During pregnancy, as the uterus expands to accommodate the growing baby, the space for the lungs decreases. This can make the breath strained and it can take more effort to activate the diaphragm each breath. The spaces between the ribs can also decrease, creating compression in the upper body. The lungs both change shape and move into a more upward direction as the baby grows.

Breathing through each asana with awareness can assist in softening the intercostal muscles between the ribs and maximise the space for each breath. Practising breath exercises can also build awareness of the movement of each breath into the body and encourage the conscious expansion of the body.

My Osteopath shared this story from when he was studying a

specialised pregnancy-related program in the USA. The professor asked the group of students, "Tell me, what is it that makes space within a woman through pregnancy?" People came up with all sorts of answers: "the movement of the internal organs", "the pushing of the lungs", "the changing shape of the ribs" and so forth. His answer was not physical but "unconditional love and sacrifice". It is that sacrifice and that love that creates space for new life.

A beautiful way to either start or finish a pre-natal yoga class is to have the students place one hand on their baby and their other hand on own heart. Mindfully, with each deep breath, feeling the expansion and release through their body and baby, while deeply connecting to baby within. Being aware of what they are giving and also what they are receiving.

Pranayama Practice

Ideally, pranayama is practised in a comfortable seated position, with a straight spine and the eyes closed. There is the option to sit in a chair or stand if necessary. Breath awareness can also be practised in a side-lying position.

During pregnancy, avoid breath retention; the growing baby needs a continual flow of oxygen from the mother. Start and finish each pranayama practice with breath awareness. The body then gets time to absorb the benefits of the breath work and this quiet time also allows for some reflection before opening the eyes.

Breath Awareness

Benefits

Can be a way to remain centred or return to centre if the mind deviates. Helps people breathe abdominally with their diaphragm. Increases awareness of the centre of gravity in the lower abdomen and base of spine.

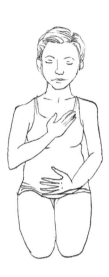

Regular practice along with building awareness of the breath creates an anchor point through labour.

How to

Breathing is not a technique, rather an involuntary rhythm. There is no need to try. There is no need to push down on exhalations, which can be damaging to the pelvic floor, nor pull in on inhales. Allow the breathing to happen normally and develop naturally over time.

In the last month or two of pregnancy, women may prefer to exhale through their mouths. This is great preparation for labour, where women's natural tendency is to breathe out through the mouth.

In a seated or kneeling position, place the left hand on the heart and the right hand on baby. Close the eyes and feel the deep connection to baby, becoming aware that each breath is also massaging and nurturing the baby inside.

Take the awareness to their breath. Ask them to notice each inhale and each exhale, feeling the movement of their hands through the chest and abdomen with each breath. Ask them to feel how their spine naturally lengthens with each breath, down towards the roots with each exhale, and up towards the head with each inhale.

Diaphragmatic Breathing

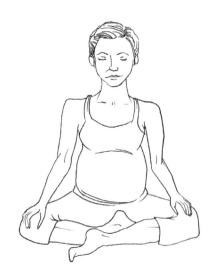

Benefits

A grounding breath that uses the whole lung capacity (base, thoracic and cervical). Engages the diaphragm fully for each breath which activates the parasympathetic nervous system.

How to

From a seated position, focus on an exhalation and empty the lungs slowly from the top downwards. As you do this, become aware of the three areas of the lungs: cervical, thoracic and abdominal region. There is a slight pause at each section, without holding the breath. Passively inhale and repeat this five times, building awareness of the exhalation.

Next, work with the inhalation. Imagining a balloon filling up, breathe in from the base upwards. Feel the air fill the abdominal region, the thoracic region and finally the cervical region, without tensing or hunching the shoulders.

Exhale fully without force, feeling the spine lengthen as the hips and pelvis ground into the earth. Repeat this cycle five times.

Now bring awareness of the full three-part breath on both the exhalation and the inhalation. Repeat ten times. Then soften through the breath and sit quietly with eyes closed for as long as desired.

Balancing Breath

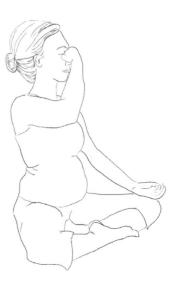

Benefits

A calming breath that balances the left and right sides of the brain. Settles the nervous system and invigorates the internal environment of the body.

How to

When practising this pranayama, it is important to let their fingers touch nostrils lightly as they alternate and close each nostril gently. Pushing too hard can create extra tension.

Using the right hand, place the thumb of the right hand beside the right nostril and the middle finger of the same hand beside the left nostril.

Begin by closing the right side with the thumb while the left nostril is kept open. Inhale through the left nostril. Without holding the breath, close the left nostril with the middle finger, release the thumb over the right nostril and exhale through the right nostril. Now close the right nostril and exhale through the left. This is one round of breath.

Follow this rhythm for at least ten rounds, or more if desired, keeping a calm and steady flow of breath.

Cooling Breath

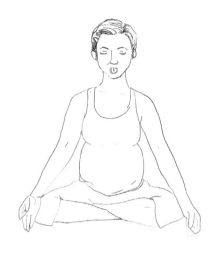

Benefits

A cooling breath that can alleviate the common discomfort of heat in pregnancy, from the additional blood volume. Through labour, birthing women can have temperature fluctuations and so practising this can help when feeling overheated.

How to

Stick out the tongue and roll the tongue. Inhale through the space in the tongue being aware of the cool air coming through the mouth. Gently close the lips and exhale through the nose.

If unable to roll the tongue, gently press the upper and lower teeth together and separate the lips as much as is comfortable, exposing teeth to the air.

Inhale slowly through the gaps in the teeth and focus on the hissing sound of the breath. Close the mouth to exhale through the nose.

Continue in this pattern of inhales and exhales for 10-20 breaths and then resume breath awareness.

Humming Breath

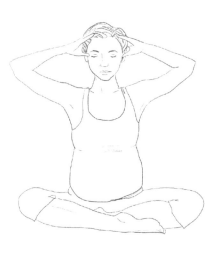

Benefits

A way to block out the surrounding distractions to move deeper within and calm the mind.

Helps extend the breath to its natural limits and overcome any partial breathing habits. Relaxes through the jaw which is necessary through labour.

Gives people permission to make sounds and noises and to practise doing something they may not normally do.

How to

In a comfortable seated position, with eyes closed, cover the ears with the thumbs and rest the fingers on the forehead and crown of the head. With the lips closed for the entire length of the exhalation, make a medium pitched humming sound in the throat. The sound is like a humming bee! Notice the gentle vibration through the mouth and throat; and the relaxation that follows through the jaw.

Do the practice for 10 rounds and when finished, return to breath awareness.

Chapter ELEVEN

Birth

Stay Focused and Stay Centred

Before the birth of my first son, I was an advertising executive with a busy, high pressure job. At that time, I thought I was in control because I met my budgets and deadlines. By feeling that I was in control, I was able to stay focused and keep achieving in the midst of the chaos that surrounds magazine publishing.

In my first labour I tried to stay in control to keep calm... which proved difficult and ultimately unrealistic for me. I couldn't control the force of labour and my centre was hard to find. My habitual way of staying centred, through thought and intellect, did not work in labour because my thinking area of the brain had to release for labour to progress.

Being centred and being in control are often confused; people try to stay in control to remain centred. Sometimes labouring women also try to control themselves by not making noises, by holding their breath or by not moving naturally because they have a fear of making others' uncomfortable. Ultimately, control needs to be released for labour to establish. A labouring woman ideally stays in her centre through the process.

There is a certain kind of chaos that a cyclone or hurricane can cause as it follows its path. In this kind of storm the safest place to be is in the centre, the eye of the storm. As the intensity of labour builds, a storm can be going through a woman and the safest place for a birthing mother is in her centre. Finding the centre and differentiating that with perceived control is one of my favourite themes for a dedicated prenatal yoga class.

In a prenatal yoga class, we can use asana as a powerful way to teach the concept of remaining centred. Repeating these asana, and having women hold the position for the time of a typical contraction, allows them to deepen their inner exploration and notice any aversions that may come up for them. 'Holding the space' to explore what happens when faced with discomfort often results in a storm of emotions inside. Asana for staying centred and staying focused include: arm circling, hitchhiker arms, toes sit, and squats.

When practising these asana, try to stay in the asana for the whole time. Take a short break if needed but encourage women to return as soon as possible.

Labour

A range of physical, mental and emotional processes unite with birth. With spontaneous labour, contractions may begin or the waters may break. In an induction, labour begins in hospital once the decision is made to induce. For cesarean, birth begins when in the hospital.

Although epidurals and birth by cesarean restrict some of the yoga practices, all births have physical, subtle and causal considerations.

The physical considerations include:

- The location where women are giving birth and the surroundings, who will be present, and who their caregivers are.
- The distance of travel to the planned place of birth from home.
- Any medical conditions they may have.
- How the body has coped with the pregnancy, and any limitations to movement, including epidurals.
- Physical elements of the yoga practice include: asana, pranayama, meditation and visualisation practices.

The *subtle considerations* include the emotional shifts and changes through birth. One sign that labour is imminent is there is an emotional release. It is as if that release opens the space for the release of baby into the world. Many women laugh with understanding when I mention this, as there are generally many emotional releases throughout pregnancy. There are often waves of different emotions. Women in labour can go from being fearful to joyful or even ecstatic in a moment. She may move from feeling angry to absolutely elated... or she may experience sadness and tears.

Causal considerations are diverse, and indeed birth can be a spiritual experience. Women may experience a deep silence within, spiritual awakenings and realisations, as she discovers her mother within. For some women, it is completely normal to not experience this. Each woman's experience of birth is unique and it is important to accept and allow all experiences. As a yoga teacher, there is a responsibility to not make promises that if women practise or breathe properly or move properly they will get a certain outcome. There are many factors involved in birth and so many variables will decide how each birth unfolds. From the yoga practice, women do build up an awareness inside and out, and this can powerfully lead them on their path through birth.

The Stages of Labour

For the purposes of this book, the stages of labour have been segment-ed into three sections: pre-labour, active labour and birth of baby and placenta. The physical, causal and subtle considerations are explored in detail in relation to these stages.

Pre-labour

In this stage, the waters may break before contractions start and there may be a bloody show. Dilation is from 0-3 cm and contractions are often irregular, but they may happen every ten minutes. The duration is not steady and one contraction may be 30 seconds, the next 45 and of varying times as the labour is trying to establish.

This period includes any induction preparation or the preparation before a cesarean.

Physical Considerations Pre-labour

As labour is starting to establish, active positions are ideal. The focus is on movements that are efficient and not too tiring as labour can go for unexpected lengths of time. Work with gravity to support baby's descent, the opening of the pelvis, and to optimise circulation.

Oxytocin flows in the bloodstream. Movement increases the amount of blood pumped around the body.

Partners can play an important role in establishing labour in the pre-labour time through their love and involvement. Oxytocin pro-duction is supported with touch, eye-contact and love, which can be given through and between contractions in various ways. That feeling of safety can reduce stimulation of the neo-cortex.

Asana for Pre-labour

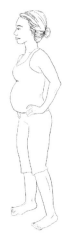

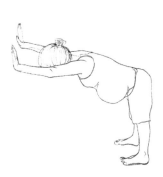

*Circling hips (can also
be on a fit ball)*

*Modified down dog (with
or without partner)*

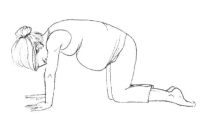

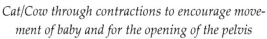

*Cat/Cow through contractions to encourage move-
ment of baby and for the opening of the pelvis*

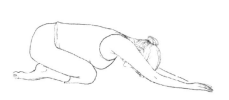

Child's pose

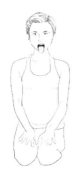

Lion's breath to release tension

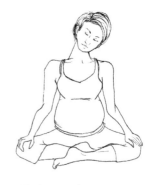

Neck stretches to encourage
relaxation through the shoulders

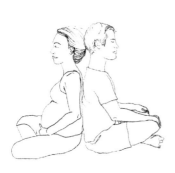

Back to back breathing

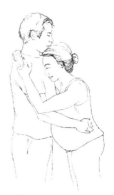

Partner sway

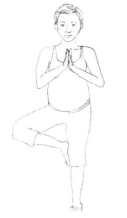

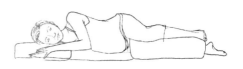

Side lying - resting between contractions

Tree pose - to return to centre

Subtle Considerations Pre-labour

There is often excitement and anticipation as the long-awaited labour shows signs of beginning. Emotions may oscillate between joy and fear. Happiness they will meet their baby soon... to worry that they are going to meet their baby soon. First time mothers might wonder if they are actually in labour yet, which can occupy their minds at times. She may worry if they will have enough time to get to the hospital (if that is where they plan to give birth) or how she will cope with contractions while sitting in a car. For women in their first labour, they may wonder how strong the contractions might become as labour progresses.

Causal Considerations Pre-labour

The time of early labour is where women might do things before having to focus solely on labour. For example, maybe a walk or swim depending on the circumstances, perhaps a sleep, or watching a movie with their partner.

Some women like to bake their favourite recipe at this time to keep distracted. A client once told me that the advice she was given was to start baking cookies when contractions began and keep going with the baking until the cookies start burning. When they start to burn, it means you are unable to focus on the cookies anymore and active labour has begun.

Active Labour

Contractions are regular and cervical dilation goes from 4-10 cm. Included here is the transition stage, which is often when the most intense contractions are experienced. At that time, contractions can last for a minute or more and be a minute apart.

Physical Considerations – Active Labour

Contractions strengthen and lengthen, which can be physically and mentally challenging. During contractions, movements that conserve energy and that assist the baby's descent are ideal through this part of labour.

Deep sacral pressure and physical support through touch during contractions not only soothes but also helps release back muscles to open the pelvis for birth. It's important to relax through the pelvic floor and allow the contractions to flow without tension through other parts of the body.

The active labour stage can become tiring and so there is usually a need for deep rest between contractions. The rest time between contractions is as important as the contractions themselves, when there is stillness to prepare for the next contraction. Child's pose or a supported wall lean are wonderful positions to take rest. Being in the shower can be a natural pain relief.

How long it has been or hasn't been may become a focus at this stage. Women might wonder if they can keep going and have the energy for it. Labour time is unpredictable and unknown. When I think about time, I like to think about the Ancient Greeks who had two words for time: kairos and kronos. *Kairos* is when we participate in time and therefore lose our sense of time passing; we are totally absorbed and in the moment. *Kronos* refers to measured time. It's what we usually mean when we think about time—clock time. In labour, the preferred place to be is in kairos. Better to be in the moment, because we never know when full dilation will happen and the labour will shift to pushing stage.

Asana for Active Labour

The following asana options for the second stage are not limited to this, just ideas from what I have observed and experienced of women moving through this stage of labour.

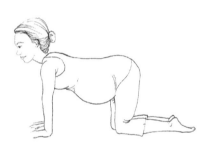

Cat/Cow, hands and knees position (supported and unsupported)

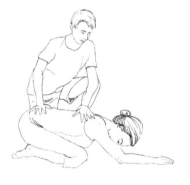

Supported child's pose

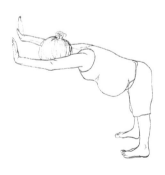

Modified down dog (with or without partner)

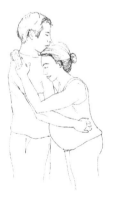

Partner sway

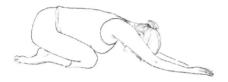

Child's pose

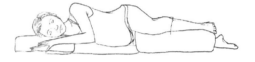

Side lying position

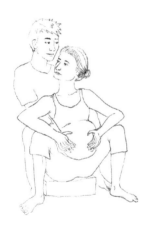

Supported partner squat

Subtle Considerations – Active Labour

Through labour, emotions can be unpredictable. Along with the flow of hormones, women can also become very tired. Women who are generally quiet may have loud and emotional outbursts and vice versa. As the neo-cortex releases, women lose their language. Women move deeply within and may also speak in unfamiliar ways. The part of the brain that profanities come from seems to be different to other language and this is why women may swear uncharacteristically in this stage of labour.

The transition phase is between 8-10 cm dilation. This time can push women well beyond what they thought their limits may be.

Causal Considerations – Active Labour

As a birthing woman moves deeper into her labour, she is on her unique journey. Also referred to as a rite of passage, through the journey great challenges are faced and transformation ultimately occurs. On the path of birth, women can often access deep places that they may not have touched on before. They discover hidden strength and new understandings.

As the contractions strengthen towards full dilation, women often release their expectations of what birth was going to be like, and with that, surrender fully into the force of nature that is birth.

Birth

Within this stage is the active pushing and birth of baby and the placenta. The cervix is fully dilated. There is sometimes a brief pause in contractions as the body shifts gears and readies to push. Often women will experience an overwhelming urge to push, which can be similar to a feeling that they need to empty their bowels.

Physical Considerations – Birth

When the cervix has fully dilated, the contractions change. Different breath and movements are experienced spontaneously through the birthing stage. The sounds women make at the pushing time differ to the dilation phase. Often women feel the urge to push.

Practise and be familiar with all the different positions because until birth, there is no way of knowing what position someone will actually birth in. When I have been present as a Doula, I have noticed women know instinctually what position they want to birth in. The position of baby, where the birth is taking place, tiredness of mother, and if any drugs have been used can all influence the possibilities. If a woman has had an epidural she will most likely need to give birth lying in the supine position. Epidural technology is constantly advancing though, and some hospitals allow side-lying position.

Quite often, second or subsequent births for a women have a quicker pushing stage as the pelvis has expanded in the past and her body has the experience of what to do in birth. I remember clearly a birth I was booked to doula for. I received the call at 6am to go to my client's house. This was her second baby. Ten minutes later I received another call to meet them at the hospital. Baby had been born in that ten minutes right there in the kitchen, with her husband on the phone to the ambulance service.

Positions for Pushing/Birth

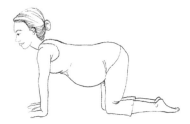

Hands and knees

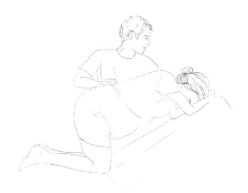

Kneeling and supported by a bean bag/ball/person/bed head

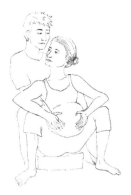

Squat/Supported squat (be aware of pressure on the perineum)

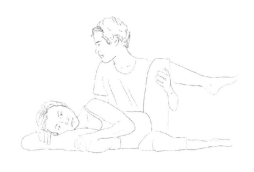

Supported side lying

Subtle Considerations – Birth

Women may cry, laugh, scream or go deeply within to birth. The emotional rollercoaster of the dilation phase generally softens here and a different set of resources need to be accessed to birth baby.

Women wonder if they will have the energy to push, especially if the labour has already been quite long. More people are in the room and there is often sporadic or continual fetal monitoring. Some women get a slight break in contractions.

Often fear arises at this stage, which can help release the adrenaline for birth.

When I think of fear in birth, I am reminded of a friend of mine who had fully dilated at home and arrived at the hospital to birth. Her pushing stage had been going for a couple of hours when she heard someone mention that they may need forceps. She said that jolted her, and from that shock and fear, she suddenly found the inner resources to birth her baby in the next couple of contractions. I have heard midwives and obstetricians speak of similar experiences.

Causal Considerations – Birth

Women can experience a wide range of spiritual experiences as they birth their baby. It is a deeply sacred space and each person will experience it in their own way. I remember when my first son was born, I had a moment of deep understanding of the purity of every single human being. That moment fundamentally changed the way I have seen all people ever since. A friend of mine told me that when her son was born she had a deep understanding of the oneness of everything. It was profound for her and life changing. Others may just be pleased that labour is over! All experiences are valid and can be validated.

Chapter TWELVE

The Fourth Trimester – Postpartum

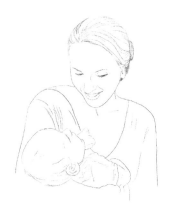

Early Postpartum

The fourth trimester is the first three months when the baby transitions from womb to world. Such major development, learning and change happens with babies in this time, and also the mother, father and family.

Not a lot of planning can be done, indeed it is surprising how this little person can take up so much time. It is usually with a first baby that the most significant relative change happens because everything is brand new.

Even with all the planning in the world, how new babies come in and affect lives is completely unpredictable. Living in the moment is one way to build resilience, and is usually where a yoga practice benefits new mums the most. Having awareness of the self when a baby is crying can be the difference between sinking into a state of helplessness and breathing through the panic, staying balanced and centred.

New mums are usually exhausted and they themselves are coming back together after the birth. This happens on the physical, emotional and spiritual planes. When I am working with pregnant women, we talk about the postpartum period and how it can go on for two to three years. Releasing an expectation of returning to a state of normal can also help with recovery and acceptance.

One curious thing is that although having a baby is a monumental and life-changing event, many women decide during pregnancy that for them nothing is going to change in their lives when their baby comes. They won't be doing what they have seen many others doing and be controlled by the baby. The baby will fit in with them. I naively thought this through my first pregnancy and I was quickly awoken to my new reality.

After my first son was born, I was moving interstate and had the task of packing up the house. In hindsight, the timing was not great, but that packing up of my house projected me forward to where I needed to be. I had a small bookshelf of books next to my breast-feeding chair and an empty box next to the bookshelf. It took me two weeks, with my newborn nearby, to get those books off the shelf and into the box. There was always something else to do, shower or sleep or feed, change nappies and clean. Time shifted for me in a non-linear way.

A recent German study found that people's happiness decreased in the first year of a new baby's life[28]. The decrease in happiness was greater than a decrease in happiness post divorce, or unemployment.

These results reflect the reality of the stresses that a newborn can bring. Stresses which include: sleep depravation, worry about the baby and the future, financial concerns, and the list can go on. Rather than candy-coating the first year of a baby's life, it can be helpful for new mothers to have the challenges normalised and to learn coping practices.

The postpartum yoga practice includes asana to help the body heal, strengthen and release stress. Meditations and breath practices can be practised throughout the day. The supportive environment of yoga classes can help to re-centre and energise new mothers. It is sometimes the community aspect and belonging to the group that is of the greatest benefit.

Before starting a postnatal yoga practice or having women return to their regular yoga classes post birth, there are a two key areas to check on. Abdominal separation (outlined below) and pelvic floor awareness (chapter five) are critical. Thus slowly building strength and awareness greatly assists the whole body through this time. Women need to seek professional help if they have issues with either.

Wait until at least six weeks' post birth and after the six-week check—performed by their caregiver, doctor or midwife—before resuming yoga asana. Relaxin is still at high levels and the bones of the pelvis and ligaments through the body are healing and coming back together. Meditation, awareness through breath, and pelvic floor exercises can be continued through or started immediately post birth.

Abdominal Separation

The following instructions are how to check for abdominal separation. By teaching postpartum students how to check separation for themselves, they can simultaneously monitor their own bodies for any changes.

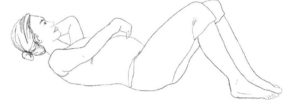

Lie in a supine position with the knees bent, hip-width distance apart, with soles of the feet on the floor. Place one hand behind the head and the other hand on the abdomen, with fingertips across the midline, parallel with the waistline at the level of the belly button.

With the abdominal wall relaxed, gently press fingertips into the abdomen. While doing this, roll the upper body off the floor into a 'crunch', making sure that your ribcage moves closer to your pelvis. Move fingertips back and forth across the midline, feeling for the right and left sides of the rectus abdominis muscle. Test for separation at, above, and below the belly button by seeing how many fingers fit into the space. Anything above two-finger-width is considered to be separation. So this needs to be addressed when doing any kind of exercise, including yoga.

To reduce separation, the transverse abdominis needs to be strengthened first.

A meditation to embrace the moment

Keep eyes open for this meditation and sit on the floor or in a chair cradling your baby. With your eyes open, softly gaze at your baby, and as you do so, soften through your breath. Keep your gaze soft and as you inhale, breathe in all that you see. As you exhale, breathe that which you see through each part of your body. With each breath, connect and embrace your baby and yourself. Motherhood is a journey and with each breath be in that moment with your baby. There will be times you love it and times you may not. Times of joy and times of sadness. Be with each emotion and breathe.

APPENDIX
Sequence Ideas

Pregnancy Sun Salutation

This is the typical sun salutation I use in my prenatal classes. I like to focus on opening up through the shoulders, movement with breath and to warm up people's bodies with some flowing movement. People connect to their breath through the sun salutations and this helps them throughout their practice. You can be creative and add variations for your own sun salutations and add some variety to the flow of the class.

Some pregnant women find the up-down movement makes them dizzy or nauseous, so before starting sun salutations, I remind women that if they start to feel dizzy or tired, take time out in child's pose until they want to rejoin the flow.

Mountain pose with feet hip-width distance apart

As you inhale, raise arms above the head

Exhale, hands down and fingertips touch
on the mat, and step left leg back

Inhale, raise arms up above the head in
lunge with the left knee on the mat

Stay here for one full exhalation and inhalation

Exhale, step left foot forward to mountain pose with arms by side

Inhale, raise arms above the head

Exhale, hands down and fingertips touch
on the mat, and step right leg back

Inhale, raise arms up above the head in lunge,
with the right knee on the mat

Stay here for one full exhalation and inhalation

Exhale, step right foot forward to mountain pose with arms by side

This is one round.

For the first sun salutation, I move slower than moving breath by breath, so students can become familiar with the flow and find the right alignment.

Repeat this sequence up to six times. If you are teaching a prenatal yoga series, students become familiar with the sequence and can flow with their breath without too much guidance after a couple of classes. Having the silent flow can allow for deep introspection and internal connection.

Sun Salutation Options

Add in cat/cow and/or down dog on each side after the lunge, for a more dynamic class.

75 minute Base Class

Sequence Ideas for a Dedicated Prenatal Class

You may have students from all trimesters in one class and it is possible to work with all of them together. The simple sequence below gives a good foundation when planning a prenatal class.

If you are teaching a class for casual students, you need to be ready to change your sequence, depending on who is in the class and what special considerations may be required.

These sequences are simply to give ideas. Work with the style of yoga you know and teach, and sequence to fit your style. It is better to avoid too much up and down motion when teaching pregnant students. Transition from standing to the mat and from the mat to standing needs to be done with care. There is never any jumping motion in prenatal yoga or strong abdominal seating. To stand up, it is more supportive to place both hands on one knee in a modified low lunge position.

The following sequence is a base class sequence I use when teaching a prenatal class. If the class is only 60 minutes, I remove some of the asanas, depending on who is in the class and if there are any contraindications for the students.

For your sequencing, add or remove asanas and time spent in each position based on the length of your class. Time for instruction and getting in and out of the positions has been included in the timings of each segment.

Squats are the 'stay in asana' for this series. Choose from the variety of squat options in the asanas section to modify the sequence.

Sequence Ideas for a Dedicated Prenatal Class

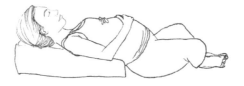

3 minutes *in Supported Reclining Butterfly*

3 minutes *Seated warm ups*

5 minutes *Hands and Knees*

5 minutes *Child's Pose twist*
& Child's Pose

Transition to standing

2 minutes *Squatting*

10 minutes *Modified Sun Salutations*

10 minutes *Standing*

2 minutes *Squatting*

Transition to seated on mat

10 minutes *Seated*

5 minutes *Back-bending*

5 minutes *Hips*

5 minutes *Legs up wall*

5 minutes *Pranayama*

5 minutes *Savasana*

Sequence for Practitioners with Pubic Symphysis

If suffering from Pubic Symphysis, care needs to be taken to manage the symptoms and reduce the likelihood of the condition worsening. This sequence offers as a way to continue with yoga to prepare for birth. Care is taken to avoid one-legged positions, deep hip and pelvis opening and squats. Place feet no wider than hip width distance apart for the standing asanas.

5 minutes *Diaphragmatic Breathing in kneeling position*

2 minutes *Neck stretches in kneeling pose*

2 minutes *Cat/Cow (keep legs as close together as possible)*

Slowly transition to standing

2 minutes each side *Standing Side Stretch*

1 minute each direction *Hips Circling*

2 x 2 minutes *Modified Down Dog at wall*
(rest in between)

1 minute each side *Standing Chest Opener*

Transition to kneeling

1 minute each side *Toe Sit with Garudasana arms*

3 x Lion's Breath in Thunderbolt

2 minutes *Hitchhiker Arms*

5 - 10 minutes *Side-lying Savasana, with no prop between the legs.*

About the Author

Gabrielle Earls is a qualified yoga teacher, doula and remedial massage therapist who specialises in pregnancy. Her work in prenatal yoga was inspired following her pregnancy with her first son in 2006.

Gabrielle has been a yoga teacher since 2008. She continually updates her training and knowledge with respected mentors and yoga teachers in Australia and internationally. She is recognised as a prenatal yoga educator through Yoga Alliance (yogaalliance.com) and certified to teach the internationally-recognised 85 hour prenatal teacher training qualification. *Birth in Awareness* is her yoga school and is a recognised Registered Prenatal Yoga School.

Gabrielle is a mentor and certified doula through *Birthing from Within* (birthingfromwithin.com). She has trained with Pam England, whose philosophy influences the work she does within the areas of pregnancy and birth.

Gabrielle lives in Sydney, Australia, with her wonderful partner and two sons.

End Notes

1. Birth & death rates | Ecology global network, 2010

2. Hytten, F. (1985) 'Blood volume changes in normal pregnancy', Clinics in haematology., 14(3), pp. 601–12.

3. *The spark of life!* Northwestern (2011) 'Radiant zinc fireworks reveal quality of human egg'. Available at: http://www.clp.northwestern.edu/news/radiant-zinc-fireworks-reveal-quality-human-egg (Accessed: 15 August 2016).

4. Marieb, E.N. and Hoehn, K. (2010) 'Human anatomy and physiology'. 8th edn. San Francisco: Benjamin-Cummings Publishing Company, Subs of Addison Wesley Longman. p.83

5. Marieb, E.N. and Hoehn, K. (2010) 'Human anatomy and physiology'. 8th edn. San Francisco: Benjamin-Cummings Publishing Company, Subs of Addison Wesley Longman. p.1075

6. Marieb, E.N. and Hoehn, K. (2010) 'Human anatomy and physiology'. 8th edn. San Francisco: Benjamin-Cummings Publishing Company, Subs of Addison Wesley Longman.p.1088

7. Marieb, E.N. and Hoehn, K. (2010) 'Human anatomy and physiology'. 8th edn. San Francisco: Benjamin-Cummings Publishing Company, Subs of Addison Wesley Longman. p.2

8. Marieb, E.N. and Hoehn, K. (2010) 'Human anatomy and physiology'. 8th edn. San Francisco: Benjamin-Cummings Publishing Company, Subs of Addison Wesley Longman. p.1089

9. Li, H., Zhou, J., Wei, X., Chen, R., Geng, J., Zheng, R., Chai, J., Li, F. and Jiang, S. (2016) 'MiR-144 and targets, c-fos and cyclooxygenase-2 (COX2), modulate synthesis of PGE2 in the amnion during pregnancy and labor', 6.

10. Marieb, E.N. and Hoehn, K. (2010) Human anatomy and physiology. 8th edn. San Francisco: Benjamin-Cummings Publishing Company, Subs of Addison Wesley Longman.

11. Marieb, E.N. and Hoehn, K. (2010) 'Human anatomy and physiology'. 8th edn. San Francisco: Benjamin-Cummings Publishing Company, Subs of Addison Wesley Longman. p.386

12. Wilson, A. (2014) 'Scientific research: How yoga works'. Available at: https://yogainternational.com/article/view/scientific-research-how-yoga-works (Accessed: 15 August 2016).

13. Marieb, E.N. and Hoehn, K. (2010) Human anatomy and physiology. 8th edn. San Francisco: Benjamin-Cummings Publishing Company, Subs of

Addison Wesley Longman.p 600

14. Uvnas-Moberg, K.U. (2011) 'The oxytocin factor: Tapping the hormone of calm, love, and healing'. London: Pinter & Martin.

15. Dick-Read, G. (2013) 'Childbirth without fear: The principles and practice of natural childbirth'. 2nd edn. London: Natl Book Network, p.38.

16. Odent, M. (2007) 'Birth and breastfeeding: Rediscovering the needs of women during pregnancy and childbirth'. 2nd edn. London, United Kingdom: Clairview Books, p.40.

17. Marieb, E.N. and Hoehn, K. (2010) 'Human anatomy and physiology'. 8th edn. San Francisco: Benjamin-Cummings Publishing Company, Subs of Addison Wesley Longman.p.1043

18. Marieb, E.N. and Hoehn, K. (2010) 'Human anatomy and physiology'. 8th edn. San Francisco: Benjamin-Cummings Publishing Company, Subs of Addison Wesley Longman. p.1044

19. Dick-Read, G. (2013) 'Childbirth without fear: The principles and practice of natural childbirth'. 2nd edn. London: Natl Book Network.p.29

20. Odent, M. (2009) 'The functions of the orgasms: The highways to transcendence'. United Kingdom: Pinter & Martin

21. Bani, D. (1997) 'Relaxin: A pleiotropic hormone', General Pharmacology: The Vascular System, 28(1), pp. 13–22. doi: 10.1016/s0306-3623(96)00171-1.

22. Dehghan, F., Haerian, B.S., Muniandy, S., Yusof, A., Dragoo, J.L. and Salleh, N. (2013) 'The effect of relaxin on the musculo-skeletal system', Scandinavian Journal of Medicine & Science in Sports, 24(4), pp. e220–e229. doi: 10.1111/sms.12149.

23. Mookerjee, I., Solly, N.R., Royce, S.G., Tregear, G.W., Samu-el, C.S. and Tang, M.L.K. (2006) 'Endogenous Relaxin regulates collagen deposition in an animal model of allergic airway dis-ease', Endocrinology, 147(2), pp. 754–761. doi: 10.1210/en.2005-1006.

24. Russell, J.G.B. (1969) 'Moulding of the Pelvic Outlet', Bjog: An International Journal of Obstetrics and Gynaecology, 76(9), pp. 817–820. doi: 10.1111/j.1471-0528.1969.tb06185.x.

25. Marieb, E.N. and Hoehn, K. (2010) 'Human anatomy and physiology'. 8th edn. San Francisco: Benjamin-Cummings Publishing Company, Subs of Addison Wesley Longman.p.344

26. Marieb, E.N. and Hoehn, K. (2010) 'Human anatomy and physiology'. 8th edn. San Francisco: Benjamin-Cummings Publishing Company, Subs of Addison Wesley Longman. p.326

27. Hill, D. (2007) 'Yoga Sutras: The means to liberation'. Victoria, BC, Canada: Trafford Publishing. p.71

28. Margolis, R. and Myrskylä, M. (2015) 'Parental well-being surrounding first birth as a determinant of further parity progression', Demography, 52(4), pp. 1147–1166. doi: 10.1007/s13524-015-0413-2.

Lightning Source UK Ltd.
Milton Keynes UK
UKHW021430080121
376678UK00008B/1918